THE BATTLE I FOUGHT AGAINST HEART FAILURE, HYPERTENSION AND THYROTOXICOSIS

The Battle I Fought Against Heart Failure, Hypertension and Thyrotoxicosis

A Living Nightmare

Hedwig Taaru

To order additional copies of this book, contact:
Xlibris Corporation
0-800-644-6988
http://www.xlibrispublishing.co.uk
orders@Xlibris.com.uk

300164

Contents

Acknowledgements 7

Chapter One: The News 9

Chapter Two: All About Thyrotoxicosis...................................... 30

About the Author.. 61

Appendix 1: Thyroid Resources 63

Appendix 2: Definitions and Terms 64

ACKNOWLEDGEMENTS

First, I would like to thank the Almighty God, who guided me and gave me strength through the illness. I would also like to thank the staff of the Royal Berkshire Hospital for looking after me.

Great appreciation is due to my close relatives and friends for the continued support they gave me and my children during the difficult time. It has made us feel part of the family.

I would like to thank my General Practitioners Dr L. Dean and Dr Syed for having taken extra care of my physical health, Dr Swinburn, the Cardiology Consultant, for his special treatment, Dr El Sheikh and her team for the special treatment and support, Sister L. Taylor and her team for the cardiac rehabilitation, and Dr Gildersleve and his team for the Radionuclide Therapy.

I would also like to thank my five children for their immeasurable love, support and care, which made my recovery far easier.

Last but not the least, I would like to thank Father Dominic, my local priest, Father Richard and Father Michael, the hospital chaplains, and the late Father Frans and other religious leaders, who gave continued and extra spiritual support during difficult times.

CHAPTER ONE

The News

28 December 2007: I was on duty as usual, a long day—a fourteen-hour shift, although I had suffered from shortness of breath (SOB) on exertion for nearly seven months. After walking a mile I would feel very short of breath; and on a few occasions I also felt chest pain and weakness. When lying down, I used four pillows rather than lying down flat, to help alleviate the SOB. I often experienced ankle swelling as well. As the SOB worsened, I rushed into surgery, where my GP diagnosed me with angina. I was given a glyceryl trinitrate pump and instructed to continue with some of my previous medication and asked to stop some, such as beta blockers. I was put on perindopril, referred for x-rays and blood testing for thyroid function, including haemoglobin, urea and electrolytes, and liver function. The x-ray results showed an enlarged heart.

29 December 2007: I was doing a long day and in-charge of the shift, but it was lunchtime and I was away from the ward on my break. The phone was ringing continuously, but every one on the ward was busy giving either treatment or lunch to the patients. Eventually, one of my colleagues answered the phone and took an urgent message for me to call surgery before 7p.m. about my blood test results. It was about 3p.m. when I returned from my break and one of my colleagues said, "Oh, Hedwig! I am sorry—your GP and his secretary rang, apparently it is very urgent. You have to give him a call today not later than 7p.m., as he will be waiting for you. He won't go home until you have returned his call."

I picked up the phone, a bit confused. All I knew was that the previous day I had been told I had an enlarged heart. Had it worsened? I had been on duty and I would have felt different, although it had been a struggle just to reach my work place, which was half a mile from where I lived. I rang the surgery and asked to speak to the secretary.

The receptionist asked, "Is it Mrs. Taaru?"

"Speaking," I said.

"Oh! I am sorry we have troubled you on duty, but it was necessary because Dr D wants to see you urgently," she said. "He said it has to be today. He won't go home before he has seen you. Could you please come into the surgery before 7 p.m.?"

We had a good team, and the second in-charge of the shift was already on the other phone trying to convince the bed managers to allow me to go to the surgery and send another nurse to take over from me. It was not easy, but it was sorted out around 6p.m., and off I went, thinking of all sorts of nasty illnesses and complications varying from hepatitis B, to HIV, to extreme high blood pressure (BP), to serious anemia (I had been anemic the past few months) and many others, but not heart failure or thyrotoxicosis (overactive thyroid). Why, I do not know.

As the surgery was opposite the hospital I was working in, I only had to cross the traffic lights to go on the other side, but it seemed like twenty miles away. Eventually I arrived at the surgery and reported to the receptionist.

With a very low voice, I said, "Mrs. Taaru. I come to see Dr D."

"Oh!" she said. "Thank you for coming. We are really sorry to have troubled you at work—it's just because the doctor said he needed to see you urgently today. Please go to the first floor and take a seat while we inform him that you have arrived. It's about your bloods results, but he will take you through."

Up to that moment, the only thing going around in my mind was cancer, because I had lost hair and had precancerous cells in the past. I was losing weight, easily irritated, short of breath, and eating a lot with no weight gain. I wondered about HIV, as my husband had rushed crazily back to Africa. *Oh my, God forbid*, I said to myself. I had no one to lean on. *I am Your orphan*, I said in prayer as I was going up the lift. I thought of my precious daughter, Katarina Mwangakenandje, only twenty-three years old, and my son David, twenty years old, Patrick, eighteen years, and the twins, fourteen years—all in full-time education. *Who will look after them? Please have mercy.*

After I sat in the waiting room for five minutes, I was still short of breath, although I had used the lift. The doctor called me in and said, "Hi, Mrs. Taaru.

Good afternoon. Take a seat."

I tried to appear comfortable although it was not possible in my state of mind.

"Mrs. Taaru, I am very sorry, but I thought I should call you in today although I was told you are on duty. I thought it is very important for me to call you in urgently. I reviewed the blood test results requested by my colleague the other day, and they don't look good at all. I have to be honest with you, Mrs. Taaru, and I could not leave you just to continue with your job. I am sorry, but your thyroid function test is very high. Look at it—it is 72. The normal level is below 20. Yours is triple that. But don't worry; we will sort it out for you. That's why we are here. I will write a prescription for a medication I am sure you may have heard of as a nurse: carbimazole. It normally works well with many people. You need to start taking it today."

I felt like a ton of stone was lifted off my shoulders.

Then the doctor continued. "Thyrotoxicosis is a nasty one if not treated early. Let me quickly see if I can identify the type you have. I am just going to ask you a few questions. Feel free to tell me anything that occurs to you, Mrs. Taaru. The doctor started asking me questions. "Any sweating?"

"Oh, yes, doctor—as you can see, it is like running water." Then, automatically, I started telling him the signs and symptoms I had at that time.

When I had finished he turned the computer screen to me and asked if I wanted to see the signs of thyrotoxicosis.

I said, "Oh, yes, I am interested." Although I had been a nurse for thirty-three years, thyrotoxicosis was one of the diseases I had missed out on; that's why I could only relate the illness to cancer or HIV. When the doctor showed me the computer screen, I realised that I had every sign and symptom of thyrotoxicosis.

"Thank God it's not Graves' disease," he said. "I now need to refer you to the endocrinologists in the hospital so they can sort this out for you. They will look after you properly as you are one of their nurses," he said jokingly.

"I am actually working on their ward," I replied.

I quickly called my son David to pick me up and take me to the pharmacy to collect my medication. I said to my son, "Come on, good man," although I was hiding the tears from him. When he arrived I said, "Could you please drive to the Oracle so that I can collect these tablets I was prescribed?"

When I showed him the prescription, he could see that I was not the mother he knew. He looked shocked and worried, and asked, "Are you okay, Mum?"

I replied, "So, so. I will tell you and Katarina and Patrick when we reach home, but you make sure not to tell the twins. I will tell them later when I feel strong enough to do so as I am feeling numb at the moment."

We reached the pharmacy after fifteen minutes. I got the medication and we drove home. When we reached home, I called the other two older children. Telling them was the most difficult part of the illness, but I also did not want them to continue worrying themselves and wondering what was really going on with me. I decided I would not be so quick to talk about the illness with the twins, Hedwig and Gelasius, who were just entering their teen years.

30 December 2007: I woke up early, still SOB but determined to go to work. All I knew at that time was that I had thyrotoxicosis and was very short of breath. *It will soon come to an end,* I said to myself in silence, not knowing that it could cost me my life. I struggled to reach my workplace by foot. I did not want to scare anyone, but, as my colleagues were professionals, the first one on night duty asked, "Are you all right, Hedwig? You look so out of breath and sweating and wheezy. I noticed the other day that you have been losing weight."

This hit me hard, but I pretended nothing was wrong. "No I am on a diet."

"Then please don't take off anymore," she said. "Do you want me to make you a cup of tea?"

"No thanks, I had one before I came to work. I just want to sit down as I am too early for the shift and I am a bit short of breath."

When it was time for the changeover, everyone on duty came into the office for the start of the shift. The nurse who was handing over charge was not too pleased with my look. She said, "Are you okay, Hedwig?"

This time I said to myself, *I have to be honest with myself and those I am looking after and working with.* I replied, "Not really." Tears began falling down my cheeks.

"Okay, I will speak to you in a minute. Just calm down." After the handover, she ordered everyone else to leave the office so we could talk. She started by asking me, "Do you have a problem, Hedwig? You don't look yourself—not the Hedwig we know."

I replied, "I don't know. Apparently I have thyrotoxicosis, and that is what is causing me to lose weight. I am eating a lot but don't put on weight. I often feel shaky, and I'm sweating even in cold weather."

"Okay, do you want me to inform the bed managers so that you can go back home and arrange to see your GP or go to A&E [Accident and Emergency]?"

"Oh, no! I will be fine. It is very hard to get someone to lead the shift and since I am already here, let me try my best," I said,

"But if you are not feeling well, please don't risk it. Please inform the person who is working with you to take the lead and ask for someone to come down from another department to take over. You have to look after yourself, Hedwig. You have children to look after as well."

I said to myself, *it is true.* I took the handover and started the shift, but at around 10 a.m. I began to feel faint. I rushed to the office; luckily one of the doctors was around.

She asked, "Are you okay, Hedwig?"

I said, "No, not really. Could you please call Nurse M for me please? Tell her it's urgent. I am not well."

The doctor went to call Nurse M. I lay down on the sofa.

Soon Nurse M arrived. "Hedwig! What's going on?" she shouted. "Come on, don't collapse in my hands. Let's take a look at you. Oh, my God! The oxygen saturation is low. You look pale, Hedwig, and cyanotic as well. Let me give you oxygen. Doctor, please come help."

"No," I insisted, "I will be fine. Let the doctors continue with their work preparing for the ward round."

It took about fifteen minutes for me to get my head back. This was when I realised that it could be something more than thyrotoxicosis. Nurse M continued to monitor me. She told me that my blood pressure was very low.

I said, "I am not surprised, because it happened once before, and it nearly put me under the ground. I need to speak to my GP regarding the BP tablets; some could be stopped."

"Shall I make you a cup of tea?"

"Oh, yes—or let me try coffee, please. I don't normally drink coffee, but that will help raise the blood pressure."

The nurse brought me coffee, and I took it and sipped it.

"Take a little rest here, but please, do call if there are any changes so we can see what we have to do."

"Okay, love," I replied. "Surely something is wrong with me. This is not me. Something has to be done. I can't be on duty like this after thirty-three years. This has not happened before. I need to book an appointment with my GP."

After twenty minutes in the office I called nurse M again and spoke to her about what I thought was the right thing to do, as I was leading the shift and nurse M was the second-in-command. I said to her, "I am going to inform the bed managers and ask them if they could release me to go back home as I am not feeling well."

The bed manager on duty was not too happy to release me, but Nurse M convinced her. Eventually, it was arranged for another nurse to come from the sister unit and take over. She came, and I handed over the ward to her. I went home, but even though it was less than a mile away, I arrived short of breath. I lived in an upstairs apartment, but I was so out of breath by the time I got into the building that I sat down on the bottom step, unable to climb the stairs. I asked myself, *Shall I call 999? What should I do?* I began to have a panic attack as well. I sat there helplessly, struggling to get my breath. "Oh, God," I shouted, "help me!" I realised I had to do something or this could be my end. I took out my phone and called David. "Can you please come down?"

A woman who was passing by stopped and asked, "Are you okay?"

I said yes with a smile, and David came rushing down.

The woman could tell I was struggling. She asked, "Do you want me to call the ambulance? Or the doctor?" There were some doctors in flat 18, on the same floor as my apartment.

"Let's wait and see."

The lady opened the entry door for some fresh air and my breathing started to improve. She then left David and me. He asked, "What next, Mum?

"Just support me to go upstairs."

This was like a bad joke. I could not believe what was happening. David held my hand, speechless. Finally, he said, "Mum, let's go to A&E."

I said, "No, darling, I am much better. I think I will be all right. Let's thank God for everything. Just help me, sweetheart, to go upstairs. I don't want to trouble the people in A&E."

I convinced him, and we went slowly, step by step, up the stairs. But by the time we reached the next floor, the situation had worsened, and this time I realised I was in trouble. "This is it," I said, "Open all the doors and windows. I cannot get any air in." I threw myself on my bed, still struggling for breath. "Please put the fan on," I said, "and open all the windows. I can't breathe. Oh, my God, please help me, save me."

I could see the tears in my son's eyes.

"I will be fine, don't worry, my darling."

The incident could not be hidden from the twins. I saw one of them put the fan on, while the other one helped to open the windows. They were shocked as they saw me struggling for breath. I knew I was ill but still didn't want to admit it. All I said was, "I will be fine. This is part of a test. It will pass, as nothing is impossible for Him, the Almighty."

My other grown-up children came from their universities and learned what happened. I looked at them as they wiped off their tears; all five of them, not knowing that my tears were waiting for them to leave the room so I could sob into the pillow. But, they did not want to leave me on my own.

31 December 2007: Early in the morning my eldest boy David came into my room just to say, "Good morning, Mum." This was our golden rule, that whoever woke up first in the household would say good morning to the rest of the family. He knocked, and when there was no answer he pushed the door open, to find me kicking on/ with one leg. "Mum, Mum! Mum!" he shouted.

I could hear him shouting but had no power to respond. Thank God for giving David to come closer.

I could still hear him shouting but could not respond. He started shaking me by my shoulders. Finally he lifted me up, and that's the moment I opened my eyes. I felt confused and tired and was in my own world.

"Are you okay, Mum? What happened?"

I could not remember a thing. My son called his brothers and sisters into the room. By now I had come back to my senses. I could hear him explaining to the others how he had found me and what he had done to wake me up. This was when I realised I was very ill.

I was supposed to do a late shift. I was getting ready when my daughter looked at me. She realized I was trying to force myself, but in reality I was not well.

"She said, "Don't say you are going to work, Mum!"

I said, "Yes, love."

She said, "I am sorry, but we have seen enough. She called the manager and told her I was unable to report for work as I didn't look too well.

I had to see my GP. By this time I was exhibiting most of the symptoms except the goitre and the prominent eyes. My GP said my liver was slightly enlarged. The doctor said this was nothing major; it could be due to the medication prescribed to treat the overactive thyroid. He asked me to come back if the condition worsened.

18 January-5 February 08: I requested for my annual leave to see if I could get better with some time off. There was not much improvement, except that I didn't have the responsibility of looking after patients during this time. I was the patient and my children were the carers, looking after mum. On February 6 I started vomiting every time I ate or drank something.

"Mum, let it be checked."

I said, "It just might be a bug, I will be fine!" I continued to vomit for about a week.

15 February 2008: The condition worsened to a point where I was no longer able to tolerate it. I called the ward as I was scheduled for a late shift. "I will go and see my GP now, I have a distended tummy," I said to my senior nurse.

She replied, "No, Hedwig, go to A&E.

I said I didn't want people to think I was breaking rules because I was a nurse in the same hospital, so the right thing to do was to follow the correct channel and go to see my GP first.

She then replied by saying, "Okay then, Hedwig, but if you cannot manage please do make your way to A&E." She asked me who I was with, and I told her that I was with my elder son David. After this conversation, and before going back to my room, I booked an appointment to see my GP. I was given two options, 8 a.m. or 10 a.m. I took the early one, as I could no longer cope with the situation. My son wanted to join me for the appointment and I agreed. We walked very slowly to the doctor, my son holding me by the hand. When we arrived we signed in. The receptionist greeted us and told us to take a seat on the next floor. Because I was so out of breath and unwell we decided to take the lift upstairs.

We sat there for a couple of minutes until my GP came out and called my name. "Taaru!" My son David was frightened to go in with me, so I told him he could wait outside while I had my checkup.

"Mrs. Taaru, how can I help you, young lady?"

I told the doctor how I had been feeling, with the vomiting and abdominal pains. He asked me to lie down on the examination table while he felt for something. I guess he wanted to feel for the liver and stones, if any. After he palpated, he said, "Mrs. Taaru, I can feel some enlargement of your liver. It feels very big, and the abdomen feels very hard. But at least I could hear the movement of your intestines."

Suddenly there were many thoughts going through my mind. *Maybe an abscess . . . . Oh please, God, not the bad one!* I said to myself.

But the doctor said, "I think you may have gall bladder stones, so I need to act quickly; just a minute while I seek further opinion from the surgeons in the hospital." He picked up the phone and spoke to the bed manager. All I could hear him say is "Could you please tell them to call me back on this number? It is urgent."

After five minutes the doctor's phone rang. I heard him saying, "Dr. S, I have got one of my patients here; she is fifty-three years old with a date of birth of 25/08/1954 and is also a member of the staff in your hospital. Presented with aforesaid complains, on palpitation these were the findings: Gall bladder stone? Was recently diagnosed with a, b, c, with known hypertension.

The surgeon responded by saying, "Let me speak to the bed manager so they can move a patient who is stable, and then we will call you."

When the surgeon called back, he told my GP that he had spoken to one of the bed managers, who was told I couldn't go to the clinical decision unit (CDU) because I worked in that ward—although I did not mind being looked after by my colleagues, because at that point I only knew myself as a patient of the hospital who was very sick! I was told to go to A&E, so I called my son David to come and walk me to A&E.

We received a warm welcome. Five minutes later, the doctor requested blood tests, inserting cannulas, etc., while the nurse took the blood pressure and temperature readings. We had to wait for the blood results and needed an x-ray to guide us. The results showed an enlarged liver, fluids all over the place, and an enlarged heart. It was a scary moment. After an hour the blood results came, and most were abnormal. "Mrs. Taaru, we have to take you to the surgical ward," they said. "We will wait for the consultant, but first we need an ultrasound to confirm the diagnosis."

When the ultrasound was done it was clear that the organs had surely enlarged and had lots of fluids surrounding them. I was admitted to a surgical ward late in the afternoon. Before 6:00 p.m., the consultant came and told me to continue with the intravenous fluids and nil by mouth (IVF, NBM.). "The good news," he said, "is that it is not a gall stone, so we don't need to open your stomach to check. See you tomorrow, Mrs. Taaru."

"Thank you, doctor," I said.

But, the same evening, the situation worsened. I tried not to show signs of suffering, and put on a smile instead.

16 February 2008: On Saturday, I felt really sick but I tried not to disturb anyone, knowing that the doctors might be attending to other patients who were worse than me, and—being a nurse—I felt it was my duty to let others get help before me. The doctor then came over and said to me, "You are written up for strong painkillers, Mrs. Taaru. Just ask if you need some.

I replied, "No thank you! I'm okay for the moment."

As the time passed, I became nauseous. I was left with no choice but to ask for an anti-sickness medication, but no food.

Later that afternoon, a nurse came to me. "Mrs. Taaru, I am sorry but we are going to transfer you to H ward."

As far as I was concerned, H ward was a gynaecologic ward. I thought, *am I losing the plot, or have I not heard well? I have an endocrine illness.*

I looked at the nurse, and she said, "Oh! I am sorry; it is just because we are closing over the weekend. Don't worry, we will transfer you along with the other patients. We will reopen early Monday morning. H ward has been informed and they are expecting you."

The time came, and we were transferred to H ward. I was directed to a bay, where I found three other women. It was a bit late and the other patients were already in bed. I went straight to my bed and sat down in a chair next to it. The observations were done. My blood pressure remained on the high side, and the nurse said to me, "We have to call the doctor who is on call for you."

The doctor came after half an hour. He was a gynaecologist rather than a GP, but it did not bother me too much because I assumed a doctor knows best. He started asking me if I had been tested for HIV, hepatitis, and all the nasty ones.

This was not really what I expected to be asked, but I had no choice other than to answer his questions in an appropriate way. I said to him, "Not at the moment, but I am positive that I don't have any of these. There is nowhere I could pick any of these illnesses because my husband left in 2006, and I haven't seen him since."

Nonetheless, I was pricked by a needle and tested for hepatitis and HIV, which came back negative. I was really becoming angry, because the problem was high blood pressure.

The doctor went to the desk and wrote up a prescription for amlodipine, a type of beta-blocker, which had been stopped by my GP because it made my body retain fluids and caused my ankles to swell.

The nurse then came with the tablet. "Hi, Mrs. Taaru. The doctor has prescribed this tablet for your blood pressure because it is very high. You need to take it now."

"What is the name of the tablet, if I may know, please?" I asked.

The tablet is amlodipine. It is for blood pressure."

I said, "I can't take amlodipine because it is a beta-blocker. My GP stopped it because it was causing water retention and gave me swollen ankles. Could you please ask the doctor if he can write up my water tablets, as I feel very uncomfortable at the moment? I can't even lie down—that's why I am still sitting up. My tummy feels so distended and uncomfortable. As I was also told that my heart, liver, and lungs are surrounded by water, this might help. I have the tablets with me in my bag. I used to take them, but my GP stopped them three months ago as I did not need them."

"No, you have to take this one. That is what is prescribed."

I said to her, "No. I will not take it."

The nurse started to become really loud; that was then when I said to her, "I am a nurse in a medical ward. I am sorry to tell you, but amlodipine can't be given to someone with fluid accumulation; that would make her even worse."

I soon regretted saying that: it made her very angry. In the end I decided to take the tablet just to end the dialogue and so that the other patients could rest, as it was around 11 p.m., but I was still sitting in the chair, which did not seem to bother the nurse. She only said, "Where are your water tablets? Can I have them?" I gave them to her and she locked them up in the bedside locker and said, "I will come back to check your blood pressure now that you have taken the tablet."

"Okay, nurse, thank you," I said.

Off she went.

Around midnight, a heath care assistant came into the bay and woke up one of the patients. Her bed was opposite mine. "I need to take your blood pressure."

The patient looked at her and said, "Why?"

"Your blood pressure is very high, and we need to monitor it."

The patient said, "I've never had blood pressure problems."

"But I was told to come and do it," the carer said.

"Okay, then, do what you were told to do," the patient said.

The assistant did the blood pressure and shouted into the corridor, "120/80,"

I heard the nurse respond from the desk, "That's good. That was quick; the tablet has worked.

Knowing that the observations had been done on a wrong patient and she was recording it in my file, I said to myself, *what a ward!* But I decided to keep quiet as I had been nearly told off before.

Time passed. Around 1 a.m. I still couldn't lie down. I decided that no matter what it cost me I would fight for my water tablets. I rang the bell. I was really traumatised by the whole thing, but I tried to keep it professional. There were tears in my eyes, but I tried to put a brave face on. The nurse came, and I asked her, "Could you please ask one of the doctors to prescribe the water tablets? I think I really need them. They might help. I am so uncomfortable, believe me or not."

"Okay, Mrs. Taaru," she said. "I will do that."

"Oh, thank you, nurse!" I said.

After thirty minutes she came and said, "I spoke to one of your doctors, and they said yes, you can have the water tablets, but now is too late. You will go to the toilet all night if I give it to you now."

I said, "Don't worry, I am used to it. Let me just have it."

She gave me the tablet, and after an hour I passed gallons of urine. I was relieved and was now ready for bed, but before that I wanted to show I was not a bad patient but somebody who was ill and needed proper care. I could have taken it further if I wanted to. I rang the bell.

She came in. "Oh, what is it, Mrs. Taaru? Did you ring the bell?"

"Yes, nurse. I only wanted to know if you are still coming to check my blood pressure, or should I go to sleep now that I am better and had some fluids off?"

"Your blood pressure has been done. I was told it was 120/80."

I said, "Could you please ask your colleague whose blood pressure she has done? She should be able to tell you, because I didn't fell asleep at all, and I know that my blood pressure was not done. The last time it was done was soon after I arrived."

She went to ask her colleague, and I assume she was then told whose blood pressure had been done, because she came back and apologised and read my blood pressure. From that night until I was discharged, she was a good nurse. I learned a lot about being a patient. However, this is about how I fought thyrotoxicosis and heart failure. I could have written more about being a patient.

17 February 2008: On Sunday I looked much better, smiling as usual. I started feeling my normal self, but I was still eating nothing by mouth. Each time I asked, it seemed there was no one who could tell me how long I would be NBM, and there was no one to ask the doctor for intravenous fluid. I hadn't eaten since Friday, but I had gone through the worse. *I am a child of God,* I said to myself. *This is not the end.*

Later, the late shift nurse who was looking after me decided to give me food. I ate it up, as I was hungry and thirsty. My colleagues came to see me and offer support and prayers.

18 February 2008: On Monday, the consultant came and as he entered the bay I gave him a big smile. He said, "Well done, you look much better. I was very concerned about you on Friday. Thank God I did not rush you to the operating theatre on Friday. I would have caused unnecessary pain. The good news is we now know that it is not gall stones, and it looks like the water tablets are working. Another x-ray and two days in bed, and I will discharge you, with appointments to see two specialists, a cardiologist and an endocrinologist respectively,"

"Oh, thank you, doctor," I replied.

20 February 2008: I was discharged on Wednesday morning and my son David picked me up. When I went home everything looked well at that time.

22 February 2008: When I woke up on Friday morning, I had severe abdominal pain. I quickly picked up the phone and phoned my manager at work. I said to her, "I was meant to be on duty as agreed yesterday with your colleague, but I don't think I can make it today."

"Oh, Hedwig! What is it?" she said. "Poor thing!"

I said, "My tummy is all bloated. I just don't know. I am going to phone my GP."

"This is sad," she responded. "Why don't you go to A&E?"

"It is a good idea, but because I am working for the trust I don't really want people to think I am abusing the service. I will just go through my GP. I will be fine."

"Okay, then, Hedwig. I'll book you off. Take care."

I picked up the phone and rang my GP's surgery. The receptionist picked up the phone and asked if she could help. I told her who I was and asked if I could book a morning appointment with my GP. She said there were one at 9:15 and another one at 12:30. I chose 9:15, although it was close to that time already. David was at home, and I woke him up and said, "I am not feeling too well, my darling. I booked an appointment with the doctor. Are you able to take me there?"

He said, "Okay, Mum, but we have to walk there because I don't have the car today. It is with Kay."

I said, "Cool, sweetheart. I will dress quickly, and then we'll go when you're ready."

He also dressed quickly, although he normally takes an hour as a young man. On our way he had to hold me, but I was trying to be strong and positive. "Why don't we call a taxi, Mum, he asked"

I said to him, "There are only five minutes or so remaining—we will be there any time. Don't worry. God is Almighty," I said to him. "He always helps us."

We arrived at the surgery a bit later than I had estimated, but before the appointment time. I booked in and was told to sit in the front of the consulting room on the second floor. David asked, "Do you want me to come, Mum?"

I said, "No, I will be alright. I will call you if necessary. Just stay in the waiting room or go for a walk." I took the lift as I could not go by stairs to the second floor. There was another patient in the consulting room, and I sat until it was my time and I was called in. When I went in, the doctor said, "Morning, young lady, what can I do for you?"

I said, "Good morning, doctor. I am not feeling well. I've had epigastric pain for the past two months, which has worsened over the past two days and became severe this morning. It is more painful on the right upper right side of the stomach. I have also started throwing up when I eat something, but I have opened my bowel well, including this morning."

"Okay, let's see if we can find the problem. Could you please lie down on the examining table so I can investigate?"

I lay down on the bed, and the doctor started the investigation. With every touch there was a severe pain on the right side.

"Okay," he said. "I am so sorry, I won't touch that side any more." Then he said to me, "The only thing I can think of is either cholecystitis or peptic ulcer. Your liver can be touched as well. It feels enlarged. And you have an enlarged heart. I will have to phone the surgeons in the hospital for advice and referral. Just wait there." He picked up the phone and gave the history and the current problem and his findings. The receptionist at the hospital gave the phone to the bed manager, as they are all trained nurses with experience.

The one who took the phone said, "The surgeons are all busy at the moment as they have an emergency, but don't worry. Give me your phone number, and they will call you back as soon as one of them becomes free."

The GP did as told. It only took approximately five minutes, and a surgeon responded. The GP introduced me to him, and he said, "Oh, wait. We have to ask the bed manager and see if there is a trolley available."

Another five minutes later the GP's phone rang. This time it was about the protocol. The bed manager said, "I am sorry, doctor, but Mrs. Taaru has to go to A&E as she is a member of staff at the clinical decision unit, and for that reason she can't come to us. The surgeons will wait for her in A&E. Please send her there."

"Okay then," said my GP in a low voice.

I imagined it was better for my colleagues to look after me when I was not feeling well but in this case it was not possible. I called David to take me to A&E as he had gone a bit far for a walk. I said, "Take your time. I am okay," but I knew I was not.

He arrived after ten minutes—not bad at all—we walked to A&E. I was very well received there as most of the staff knew me there as well. They did not have a problem with looking after me. They took blood and conducted the other investigations. The junior surgeon came to see me on arrival, and as per protocol she requested a chest x-ray and intravenous fluids and nil by mouth. While we were waiting for the tests to come back I went for my x-ray. When I returned the results were back, and the senior surgeon was also in A&E waiting for me. After I was transferred to my trolley in A&E the doctors came and introduced themselves. They told me about the results and said, "The good news is, it is not cholecystitis. Neither do we think it is a peptic ulcer. But we need to take you for an ultrasound to rule this out. The x-ray still showed that your heart is enlarged. We need to investigate further. Meanwhile, you remain nil by mouth, and we are going to book the abdominal ultrasound as an emergency procedure."

After fifteen minutes the porters came to take me for the procedure. I underwent the ultrasound, and when I came back one of the doctors came to see me. He said, "Oh, good news, Mrs. Taaru! It is not what we thought. But there is also a bit of bad news: your liver and your heart are enlarged, and both these organs and your lungs are surrounded by fluids. I am not surprised because of the pain you've had over the few weeks. But we will sort it out for you. I am going to call the heart doctors to come and see you, because I think from our point of view we don't need to admit you. They have to decide." He contacted the other doctors, who did not take long to come.

This time it was the consultant cardiologist who came. He asked me all the relevant information after he introduced himself, and started with the investigations. He said, "Mrs. Taaru, we need to take you over. I will increase your water tablets and start you on a small dose of beta-blockers as your blood pressure is also on the rise, and I need to see you at the end of April as my list is overbooked at the moment—but if any changes occur in between please feel free to come to A&E. The nurses here should call me. I will come or send my colleagues to see you. For now, I will discharge you after three hours, if the nurses are happy. You can go home if there is a responsible person to look after you."

I said, "Thank you, doctor, there is someone to look after me."

After three hours I went home, and because the water tablets had been increased I had changed into a different person. I was feeling really far better as the tablets started draining the excess water out of my body. I stated to feel great.

8 March 2008: I went to see my GP because I wanted to return to work, but my manager would not let me as I had been going back and then phoning in sick after a few days. My GP did not want to take unnecessary risks, so he investigated further, after which he concluded, "You look well, not SOB at rest, but you have a tender hepatomegaly with a 5 cm palpable lobe in the epigastrium." Then he said, "Let's wait until you have seen the cardiologist and then he might decide whether to send you back to work. I'm giving you a sick note to cover the next period as I think we are in a bit of a danger zone for work."

I could not understand why it happened to me. At the end of the day I was not worse, but I was sweating profusely and continuing to thin. I kept telling those who wanted to know that I was on a weight loss program.

Some were saying, "Oh, don't take off anymore!" Others said, "Oh, you look good."

If they knew that I was going through the worst time of my life, they would probably not even ask me anything. If they only knew that I had even dropped my studies, which had been going so well and which I had thought I would complete.

I took my sick note, went home and rested.

31 March 2008: This morning I was seen by the cardiologist in his clinic, who confirmed a diagnosis of dilated cardiomyopathy, thyrotoxicosis, and hypertension

7 April 2008: After seeing me in the cardiology clinic the cardiologist decided that I needed to be off work for at least another month. He said he would review my condition in a month.

15 April 2008: The GP saw me. The concentration was on the cardiomegaly, and a further sick note was issued, along with routine medication.

29 April 2008: I was seen in the cardiology clinic. The consultant cardiologist was a bit happy this time because of the progress I had made. He referred me to the senior cardiology nurse to start with cardiac rehabilitation sessions every Tuesday and Thursdays. The same day I was also seen by the endocrinologist about the thyrotoxicosis and its treatment.

12 May 2008: I was seen in the cardiology clinic, purely for the doctor to review my progress and advice my GP on any treatment that might be needed.

21 May 2008: I was seen by my GP for further medication and a further sick note

12 June 2008: I was seen by the occupational health registrar in the Royal Berkshire hospital regarding my fitness to go back to work. A letter was send to my GP and the consultant cardiologist. Meanwhile, I continued with the sick leave

16 July 2008: I was seen in the cardiology clinic. The consultant cardiologist decided to write to my manager that she had to allow me to return to work as staying home for too long might affect my psychological health, and it might be against the Disability Act as well. I took the letter and I was told that I could come back to work as there was a shortage of staff, but only on light duty and for two weeks. I said okay, but was not too sure about this, as the ward is an emergency ward and the manager said they could not redeploy me across the hospital then.

7 August 2008: The occupational heath registrar of the hospital was happy with my progress but advised me to take it easy and slowly. He wrote to my GP and my manager and all the consultants concerned.

3 September 2008: I was seen in my GP's surgery, a bit SOB and coughing this time. He investigated and reassured me that it looked like a normal cough, but because I did have a fever I was written up for antibiotics, and further blood tests were ordered, which were done in the hospital laboratory.

25 September 2008: I was seen by my GP regarding a benign lump on the left side of neck and for review of previous blood results, which revealed longstanding abnormal liver function test and a high erythrocyte sedimentation rate and globulin. He noted that I had recently been tested for HIV and all types of hepatitis, for which I had tested negative He did not know what to do any more but referred me back to the endocrinologist to review the carbimazole, as it might be affecting the liver.

30 September 2008: My pharmacist reviewed my medications and spoke to the endocrinologist regarding carbimazole and its effect on the liver. The carbimazole was changed to another medication, propylthiouracil, which I am taking to date.

21 October 2008: I saw my GP in his surgery. He was very happy with the progress I had made and was happy to give me permission to travel, as I wanted to visit family abroad and also get some fresh air.

6 November 2008: I visited the surgery in preparation for my holiday and received an inactive influenza vaccine, Pneumovax, and was told to continue with my other medication as usual. I agreed to take anti-malaria treatment on arrival in Oshakati as per protocol of the ministry of health in Namibia.

17 November 2008: I saw a specialist in Namibia about the swollen ankles. He requested a thyroid scan, which had not been done in nearly two years since my first diagnosis. The scan revealed nodules in both lobes of the thyroid gland.

2 December 2008: I asked my GP to write to my manager, who did not want to accept my report after I changed my return flight so that I could be treated, although I had sent her an e-mail about the changes in my condition while abroad.

9 December 2008: I was seen in the endocrinology clinic and received a final diagnosis of toxic multinodular goitre, thyrotoxicosis, primary dilated cardiomyopathy, and essential hypertension. On this day I was told that a letter would be written to approach the specific surgeons dealing with thyroid to see if they could help.

6 January 2009: I was seen in the GP surgery as an emergency case due to swollen ankles and shortness of breath due to standing for a long time. I had been redeployed to work in a clinic where nurses apparently were not allowed to sit during consultation of patients, irrespective of known conditions like mine.

15 January 2009: I was seen in the GP surgery with symptoms of left leg weakness, sickness but no vomiting, and epigastric pain. I was given omeprazole for epigastric pain.

And was sent back home.

16 January 2009: I handed in my resignation as I could not stand the hassles I was suffering anymore.

19 January 2009: I was seen in my GP surgery and the endocrinology clinic for the high thyroid function test, and because I had resigned.

12 February 2009: I was admitted to the hospital due to the high level of thyroid hormones or thyrotoxicosis, primary dilated cardiomyopathy, and hypertension. I stayed in hospital until February 27. That was the day on which I said the doors had opened and my prayers had been answered. A man with a white gown came in, smiling all the way as if he already knew me. "Mrs. Taaru?" he asked.

I said yes.

He pulled back the curtains and called the rest of the team in, accompanied by the ward sister. He said, "Mrs. Taaru, I am the doctor in charge of nuclear medicine. Your doctors approached me here. I think your blood results have come down to a level I am satisfied with, and I am now ready to give you the treatment." He explained to me how it worked and that I should not fear because of my heart. The doctor and nurses would be behind the door to come in if any emergency might arise, as nobody would be allowed in after the capsule was administered. "We will transfer you to our own ward so that we can prepare you there."

"Okay, doctor. Thank you so much." I was relieved because I knew where we were heading.

Later that day I was transferred to the oncology ward. Everyone was really nice. The priest later came to see me in preparation for the treatment.

3 March 2009: Early this morning my son came to see me, as my children had been told that after the treatment, visitors would not be allowed physical contact with me. They would only be allowed in for twenty minutes and had to stay a few meters away from me.

Around 9 a.m., a physician explained the process to my son and I. He also let us know that they hadn't got the capsule yet as it was not stocked in the hospital and had to be ordered from outside. Not too long after that, around 11:30a.m., two experts came. My son then went home and left me in their capable hands. I could see the concern on his face. I said to him, "God loves us, David. Don't worry, I will be fine."

All the measures were taken and I was asked if everything had been explained to me. I said yes, and then I was asked to sign the consent before the capsule was administered. The nurses came to do the observations and put the bell within reach in case of an adverse reaction to the radioactive iodine. After the nurse had left the room the physician asked, "Are you ready, Mrs. Taaru?"

I said, "Yes; may I pray first, please?"

"Oh yes, please do."

I prayed in silence, and at this point I remembered the priest, who had said to me, "Hedwig, if God wants you to go on the other side of the river, and you have to go through a dark narrow tunnel and there is no other gate, no matter how dark it is you just have to go through it because the Almighty will be there to guide you through. Please be calm and relax; God is looking after you." After I had finished with my prayer, I said, "I am ready now."

The physician reconfirmed by asking me my date of birth and address. After this was confirmed, I swallowed the capsule under strict supervision and said, "Dear God, please help me."

Another measurement was taken and protective materials put over the toilet and bathroom floors. After that, they left the room. I stayed in the room for three days with only my bible and rosary for company. I thanked God for his mercy. I was given food behind the door. It was as if I was suffering from an infectious disease that had no cure and people were afraid that I might pass it on. But it was all for my benefit. All went well in that room as I waited until I was ready for discharge on the fourth day

6 March 2009: The doctor said I was ready for discharge. I felt good and was very happy. The doctor discharged me only after the physicians said the results were fine. I was over the moon. I could not even wait for the medication I was to take home with me. It was as if I was being released from prison. I called my daughter to pick me up. My son and daughter both came and off we went. At home, I was still confined to my room, but because this was my environment I did not worry too much. I was isolated at first from the general public and then from children under five. I was instructed to:

Avoid journeys on public transport and avoid places of entertainment for five days after discharge.

Avoid prolonged close contact with adults for 16 days after discharge.

Avoid close contact with children 3-5 years for 21 days after discharge and finally, avoid prolonged close contact with children under the age of three for 27 days after discharge.

Then, the physicians conducted a review and I was finally free to mix with the general public but avoid working with pregnant women, the elderly and very young children. I had to continue with monthly consultations with the two specialists—the cardiologist and the endocrinologist—and keep my GP informed.

22 September 2009: I visited the cardiology clinic. I was called in after about half an hour. The cardiologist looked at me and said, "Good morning, Mrs. Taaru, how are you?"

I said, "I am good."

He replied, "I can see from your body you really look good compared with the last time I saw you. Meanwhile, thank you very much for the basketful of presents. I was very much impressed to see all the things you sent us. I had to call everyone in the unit to come and see what you brought us. It was massive. I said to them at least there are people who know what to give—not always sweets. It is really much appreciated."

I said, "Oh, thank you! I also appreciate the help you guys gave to me. You saved my life."

Then he said, "Let's go back for the consultation."

He did all the observations including the weight measurement, and then he said, "Woo! You put on so much weight in just a few months."

I said to him, "I visited my family in Africa, and I was fed like a baby because the family could not believe their eyes. But, I will try to keep working on it."

In a very happy mood, he said, "You put on six kilograms since the previous occasion. Please try to work on it as much as you can—not frightening people, but in a very nice way, because we have to look after that heart." He said it in a very charming way. "Let me send you for the echocardiogram scan, and we'll see what it tells us. Just wait there. I am taking this form to the radiographers." When he came back he said, "Please just wait outside in the waiting area. They will call you in and then do the scan."

I waited outside, and my name was called after forty minutes, as they were busy that morning. The scan was done by a female radiographer, who later called the other radiographer to come and confirm the results. I could tell from the slight looks of happiness on their faces that the news was good, although they did not really want to tell me as it was the cardiologist's job to inform me. I heard them telling each other it looked normal but at the same time there was a query when they compared it to the previous scan. I thought I had to ask them because I had started becoming excited in a way. I asked them, "Are we winning?"

They both said, "Yes, Mrs. Taaru, but the doctor will tell you all about it. We will give the report to him." The report was given to him, and after fifteen minutes the doctor called me in.

You could see the happiest smile on his face. He said, "Right. This is really good. I suspect the heart failure was caused by the thyrotoxicosis, because to me the heart is more than normal for your condition and age. I don't need to see you anymore unless anything nasty comes up again, but I don't hope so. I will discharge you back to your GP. I only want you to reduce on the diuretic—the furosemide—and then stop. I will write to your GP anyway. Your blood results related to the heart are all normal. Your TSH—your thyroid-stimulating hormone—is still under, but I will have to leave that to the endocrinologist to sort out. I'd rather not get involved."

I could not believe what I heard. In my heart I started singing songs of joy and praise the Lord! I felt like running. It was a miracle: from 25-30 per cent function to 59-60 per cent. It was unbelievably encouraging. I said to myself, *I only have to fight the thyrotoxicosis and the high blood pressure! And soon both will be things of the past.*

20 October 2009: One of the endocrinologists saw me in their clinic. He also said, "Mrs. Taaru, you need to watch that weight."

I said, "I promise I will, but very slowly, as I am still trying to get my head around the miracles. But I will.

"Okay," he said. "Let's look at your blood results. They look good, but your TSH is still suppressed. I might need to give you another dose of radioactive iodine if the tablets aren't doing the job. Continue to take your medication, and we will see you next time."

Final Word

I would like us to remind ourselves that no matter what we are going through, we should not forget there is a living God. Remember the following texts from the Holy Bible, to mention just a few. They worked for me; they will for you as well: Psalms 23:1, 27:1, 50:15; Isaiah 41:10; Revelation 21:7. The next chapters will tell all about thyrotoxicosis, heart failure, and essential hypertension.

CHAPTER TWO

All About Thyrotoxicosis

Your Thyroid Gland! What is it?

Many are unaware about the thyriod gland unless they are diagnosed with a thyroid disorder It was noted that about 12 per cent of the adult population worldwide suffers from a thyroid disease. It was also noted that twenty per cent of all women will develop autoimmune thyroid disease, usually hypothyroidism, and nearly a fifth of all people over sixty have subclinical hypothyroidism or mild hypothyroidism.

The purpose of this chapter is to describe where the thyroid gland is located, what is does and how it works. It will further explain the most common thyroid disorders, their causes, signs and symptoms, and common treatments. In addition, it will also address common misinformation that sometimes interferes with the diagnosis of thyroid problems.

Location of the thyroid gland and its functions

The thyroid gland is sometimes referred to as a butterfly-shaped gland, which is also shaped like a capital H. Each side of the butterfly or H is called a lobe and the body is called the isthmus. The thyroid gland is located in the lower part of the neck, in front of the windpipe. It is basically wrapped around the windpipe.

The thyroid gland makes two important hormones: the first one is called the thyroxine, known as T4, which has four iodine atoms for each hormone molecule. The second is called triiodothyroinine, or T3, which has three iodine atoms for each hormone molecule. These two hormones are referred to in the singular form as thyroid hormone.

Thyroid Hormones and their functions

The thyroid hormones serve as the speed control for our cells, controlling their speed of life. These hormones are released by the thyroid gland in two different levels, 80 per cent as T4 and 20 per cent as T3. There is only a tiny percentage of T4 in the bloodstream (0.03) in free form, and can be taken up in a body cell to do its job effectively as a thyroid hormone.

The Pituitary Gland, its function and its relationship with the Thyroid Stimulating Hormone (STH)

The pituitary gland is situated at the base of the skull and is the most influential gland in the human body. Therefore, most of the time it is referred to as a master gland. It also acts as the body's "thermostat" because it sends out many types of stimulating hormones to the various parts of the body that make hormones.

The thyroid gland reports directly to the pituitary gland, which monitors the T4and T3 level in the body. If the levels are falling, it secretes TSH, which in turn signals that the thyroid gland must make the thyroid hormone. The TSH stimulates the thyroid to take iodine from the blood and make the thyroid hormone. If the pituitary gland is working well, a high level of TSH means there is not enough thyroid hormone in the blood. A low level of TSH means there is too high a level of thyroid hormone in the blood. Normal level of the thyroid hormone results in a normal level of TSH. The TSH level in the blood is measured in order to tell whether the thyroid is making enough, too little or too much thyroid hormone. The TSH test is regarded as the most accurate and sensitive blood test available for people who suffer from a thyroid disease.

Hypothalamus and its function

The hypothalamus is a gland located in the brain just above the pituitary gland. It is actually connected to the pituitary gland by a very thin stalk that carries hormones, which help control the pituitary gland. A part of the hypothalamus also functions like a thyroid hormone by releasing its own signal, the thyrotropin-releasing hormone (TRH) or TSH-releasing hormone, to the pituitary when the thyroid hormone levels are low. Therefore, one can say there is a double-thermostat control of the thyroid hormone in the body although this can break down when things go wrong with the hypothalamus.

Primary (Hyperthyroidism) Thyrotoxicosis

It is when the disease is within the thyroid gland.

Secondary Hyperthyroidism

It is when the thyroid gland is stimulated by the excessive thyroid-stimulating hormones in the blood.

What is a thyroid gland?

The thyroid gland is an organ that is considered to be a part of the endocrine system. The endocrine system is made up of different glands, which are located in various parts of the human body. These glands produce chemical compounds called hormones that are secreted into the bloodstream. Hormones travel to different organs and tissues and exert actions that help regulate the body's metabolism, the chemical balance, and the reproduction function.

There are also other glands that are considered to be part of the endocrine system such as the ovaries, the testicles, pancreas, adrenaline glands, pituitary gland and the parathyroid glands.

Thyroglobulin and its function

Thyroglobulin (Tg) is a specific protein made only by the thyroid cells or thyroid cancer cells, and is mostly used by the thyroid gland to make the thyroid hormone. Thyroglobulin also plays a role in the treatment of thyroid disease as a screening marker of thyroid cancer recurrence. This means that after the thyroid gland has been removed, because of thyroid cancer, thyroglobulin should not be manufactured anymore. If this protein happens to be found in a blood test after the thyroid is removed, it indicates that thyroid tissue has remained and could be a sign of recurrent thyroid cancer.

The Calcitonin and its function

The cells that produce the thyroid hormone in the thyroid glands are called the follicular cells. The thyroid follicles are contained within the capsules of the thyroid gland like bunches of microscopic grapes. Between the neighbouring follicles are tiny blood vessels, lymph vessels and collections of other cells called parafollicular cells. These parafollicular cells or C-cells make additional hormones such as calcitonin and somatostatin. Calcitonin helps regulate the calcium and therefore helps prevent osteoporosis.

The Parathyroid Gland and its role

The parathyroid glands are usually four, although they can be sometimes be three to six glands located very close to the thyroid gland. That is why they are called para, meaning "near the thyroid". The function of these glands is different from that of the thyroid, which is to produce the thyroid hormones. The para glands produce parathyroid hormones (PTH), which is important in controlling calcium in the human body.

It also helps the kidneys retain calcium in the blood while releasing phosphorus in the urine. At the same time, it also increases the activation of vitamin D, which helps with the absorption of calcium and phosphorus from food and beverage containing these two minerals. However, this gland may be at times accidentally removed during a surgical procedure on the thyroid gland, or may even be damaged.

Where is the thyroid gland located?

The thyroid gland is located in the lower front part of the neck just below the Adam's apple and above the top of the breastbone. It is made up of two lobes, which are called the right and left lobe. These lobes are connected by a narrow band of tissue called the isthmus. A thin band of tissue called the pyramidal lobe may extend upward from the isthmus.

The thyroid gland is shaped like a butterfly with each lobe representing a wing. It wraps around the larynx and trachea that pass through the front of the neck. The lobes of the thyroid gland are tucked behind the angled muscles that are connected to the top edge of the breastbone. It is usually difficult to see the outline of the thyroid gland beneath the skin, though it may become more visible if the lobes become enlarged (called goitre).

What does the thyroid gland do?

The thyroid gland produces, stores, and secretes thyroid hormones called the thyroid stimulating hormones, which control the metabolic rate of tissue (TSH).

What is a thyroid hormone?

A thyroid hormone is a chemical compound that is produced, stored and secreted by the thyroid gland. The thyroid tissue is made up of specialised cells that are organised into spheres called follicles and are therefore called follicular cells. In a normal functioning thyroid tissue, follicular cells are stimulated by a hormone called TSH that is secreted by the pituitary gland. The TSH is also known as thyroid stimulating hormone or thyrotropin. When the TSH are circulating in the bloodstream, they bind to structures called TSH receptors located on the outer surface of the follicular cells, and stimulate them into taking up iodine from the bloodstream. The iodine that is taken up from the bloodstream by follicular cells is used to produce a thyroid hormone. There are two forms of thyroid hormone, the major one called T4 and the minor one called T3.

What do the thyroid hormones do?

The thyroid hormone is active in a number of organs and tissues through the human body. For example, during pregnancy the thyroid hormone helps regulate the development of the unborn baby's brain and central nervous system. During childhood and adolescence, the thyroid hormone helps regulate the growth of the bones and maturation through the different stages of puberty. In adults, the thyroid hormone helps regulate the body's metabolism by influencing the rate of energy consumption. It helps regulate the heart and blood vessels system called the cardiovascular system by influencing the rate at which the heart beats, the force with which the heart muscle contracts and the degree to which blood vessels constrict and relax. The hormones also help regulate the function of the gastrointestinal tract, the reproductive system, the respiratory system, and the brain and central nervous system.

What is thyrotoxicosis?

Thyrotoxicosis is when there is an increased level of the thyroid hormone in a person's blood. Thyrotoxicosis affects two per cent of the population in the United Kingdom. It is ten times more common in females. In forty per cent cases, the disease is self-limiting.

In Caucasians, it affects 2%-3% of women and 0.2%-0.3% of men. In general, thyrotoxicosis affects more women than men with a ratio of 9:1, and has been reported at 0.8 per 1000 per year in women and 0.1 in men during the follow-up period.

Types of thyrotoxicosis

Primary (Hyperthyroidism) Thyrotoxicosis

It is when the disease is within the thyroid gland.

Secondary Hyperthyroidism

It is when the thyroid gland is stimulated by the excessive thyroid stimulating hormones in the blood.

Signs of Thyrotoxicosis

There are many signs of thyrotoxicosis, but the following are the prominent ones.

Adrenaline Rush

When a person gets too much thyroid hormone in the body, the adrenaline also increases. Together with the high level of thyroid hormone, this causes the heartbeat to increase. This raised heartbeat can be controlled by prescribed beta blockers, which will help slow down the heartbeat. The beta blockers will also help prevent severe heart symptoms that can worsen the thyrotoxicosis.

Behavioural and Emotional Changes

Thyrotoxic people experience a range of emotional symptoms. They include nervousness, restlessness, anxiety, irritability, sleeplessness and insomnia. Some thyrotoxic patients became easily angry, some suffer from disordered thoughts, and some suffer from mood swings, similar to the ones in mania that is present in bipolar disorders.

Bowel movements

More frequent bowel movement than usual is mostly a sign of thyrotoxicosis. Although the stool is not liquid, it is still more often because digestion speeds up.

Easy bruising

People with thyrotoxicosis are bruised easily because the blood vessels, which are very small, are made more fragile by thyrotoxicosis. They may also have sweaty and warm palms, fine tremor, and they may have fast heartbeat called tachycardia, which could be with atrial fibrillation (AF), a common condition among the elderly.

Hair changes

People with thyrotoxicosis may have hair thinning and loss of hair, or diffused alopecia. This may make the hair difficult to style. Those with curly hair may notice that their hair becomes straighter, some notice that their hair is falling to an extent where it is found in clumps on the pillow, clothes, or on the brush while brushing the hair or combing for those who use combs.

Heat intolerance

Heat intolerance is known to be a classic sign of thyrotoxicosis. The body temperature might rise a bit in people with thyrotoxicosis but even in normal room temperature, a person with too much thyroid hormone will still feel too hot and sweat far more than usual, which results in an unpleasant combination. It makes people feel isolated in their environment and many wonder if it is really hot or is it just them. These symptoms are similar to the hot flashes of menopause in women.

Heart palpitation

One of the fist signs of thyrotoxicosis is a fast, forceful heartbeat called heart palpitation. This is because of the increased level of thyroxine (thyroid hormone) in the blood. Thyrotoxicosis also makes a person more sensitive to their own adrenaline, which further stimulates the heart rate. This is normally noticed only when it becomes severe, about 150 beats per minute. Thyrotoxic people often notice heart palpitation, especially when they are reading, sleeping, or involved in other relaxing activities. If untreated, heart palpitation may cause atrial fibrillation, a common heart rhythm abnormality although it is a very rare condition in thyroid patients. It only means that the person might have an irregular heart rhythm with random pauses and bursts of heartbeats. This, however, could be a very serious condition and is normally associated with other underlying heart conditions and needs the intervention of a cardiologist.

Heart palpitation or fast pulse may also cause congestive heart failure, which can cause swollen ankles and even a collection of fluid in the chest and shortness of breath. Thyroid-related heart problems are treated with beta-blockers that will slow down the heartbeat. Once the thyroid hormone levels are restored to normal, your heart will resume its normal rate.

Infertility

If a person has too much thyroid hormone in her body, it can interfere with her ovulation cycle and this may result in temporally infertility. But, once the thyroid levels are corrected to normal, a person should be able to conceive provided that the infertility was caused by thyrotoxicosis and not other conditions such as blocked tubes. Thyrotoxicosis in early pregnancy can lead to miscarriage and if a person had repeated miscarriage, it is advisable to consult your GP and have this checked out.

Low blood sugar

Low blood sugar has also become a common sign of thyrotoxicosis. Low blood sugar, also known as hypoglycaemia, triggers the same adrenaline-rush reaction that occurs during a panic attack. Hypoglycaemia can be measured with a special blood sugar masjien or a glucometer specifically designed to do this. When the blood sugar reading is below 50mg/dl (3.5mmol/L), it is considered too low. The problem is that both a panic attack and a true hypoglycaemic attack show rapid activation of the adrenergic system, which is enhanced by thyrotoxicosis. Therefore, thyrotoxicosis can be mistaken in panic attacks and false episodes of hypoglycaemia. Both symptoms can be relieved by beta-blockers and the correction of thyrotoxicosis, if diagnosed, will relieve the rest of them.

Menstrual cycle changes

It has became apparent that thyrotoxic women will find they had lighter periods and may even skip some periods because thyroid problems can interfere with ovulation and menstrual cycles and also affect fertility. When their thyroid hormone is restored to normal levels, their cycles should also return to normal. There may also be:

- Brisk reflexes
- Goitre prominent in neck
- Thyrotoxic goitre, which develops due to hyperthyroidism or too much stimulation of the thyroid. This causes the gland to enlarge. In extreme cases, the goitre can enlarge to the size of a grape but this is very rare. It normally swells to the size of a plum.

Eye problems

In many patients with thyrotoxicosis, eye problems are associated with the high secretion of adrenaline. This causes the eyelid to retract and is often called the thyroid stare. There are also additional eye changes called Graves' ophthalmopathy or thyroid eye disease (TED). This is more frequent in patients with Graves' disease and thyroid disorders. The muscles surrounding the eyeball may swell and cause the eyeball to protrude. The skin around the eyes may swell and finally the whites of the eye might become red and irritated.

Exhaustion

Excessive thyroid hormone in the body affects the energy level as well as general emotional wellbeing of a person, although this can also happen because a person might not get enough sleep or suffer from insomnia.

Muscle weakness, or sometimes wasting

Muscle weakness is a common sign in people with thyrotoxicosis and is especially noticeable in the shoulders, hips and thighs. This makes it impossible for people with this disease to climb stairs. The muscles might also ache or feel soft. Shoulder ache is more common when a person is brushing hair or does any other upper arm activity. Muscle weakness is also exacerbated by the worsening of arthritis or osteoporosis, or it may be due to a partially overworked and exhausted body. Nonetheless, there is good reason to believe that thyrotoxicosis has a direct effect on muscle function and can even cause muscle wasting, especially the skeletal muscle. Therefore, one must get a muscle problem checked out by your GP so that other common autoimmune diseases can be ruled out. For instance, myasthenia gravis, a condition which afflicts the muscles and causes muscle weakness.

Sexual function and libido

The effect of thyrotoxicosis differs in men and women. The important signs in women are an increased desire of sex because of the effects of thyrotoxicosis on their brain function and behaviour. On the other hand, menstrual irregularities and weakness caused by thyrotoxicosis might reduce a woman's wellbeing and sex drive. Many men, on the other hand, experience a decreased libido which seems to be related to increased signs of estrogen effects, including an abnormally enlarged breast. Some of this may be because of thyrotoxicosis, which increases the amount of sex hormone-binding globulinor protein that is made by the liver. This reduces the amount of testosterone available. This leads to many men with too much thyroid hormone complaining of impotence. Some even experience low sperm count and, thus, impaired fertility. An adolescent male who develops hyperthyroidism may experience a delay in development during puberty. Thyrotoxicosis might also have an effect on the brain function, which includes thoughts and behaviour. This might also affect their libido.

Skin changes

People with thyrotoxicosis might develop a very fine silky skin. This is due to the excessive thyroid hormone. The skin will feel moist with remarkably few wrinkles because of the prespiration and the constant moisture may cause a rash from inflamed pores. There might also be areas on the skin that darkens, particularly the palm and areas that itch. Some parts become very sensitive to touch and swell with minimal contact. You can seemingly write your name on your skin then.

Tremors

Hands that tremble have become an important and common sign of thyrotoxicosis. This means a person may feel a bit nervous and became shaky at all times. This is caused by the adrenaline like effects of thyrotoxicosis, but this sign will clear or improve when a person starts to take beta-blockers and the thyroid levels are corrected.

Weight loss

Weight loss is common in some thyrotoxic patients because of an increased metabolic rate, which itself is a result of an increased thyroid hormone. Despite the healthy appetite, many people still lose weight. Thus, overweight thyrotoxic patients find this a bonus but it should not be abused and intentional thyroid hormone overdoses must not be taken to lose weight.

People normally lose ten to twenty pounds and not all patients lose weight. Some end up gaining weight because they are at many times so exhausted and try to eat more to gain their energy and, consequently, become less active.

Thyroid storm

It has been noted that in some cases the symptoms of severe thyrotoxicosis can manifest as a storm of severe thyrotoxic symptoms. These include cardiovascular diseases where the symptoms might require emergency admission to a hospital and, sometimes, admission into an intensive care unit. However, this has become less common since the use of beta-blockers and the development of the TSH.

Fingertip and fingernail changes

In some thyrotoxic people, the fingertips become swollen to the point where they look clubbed which is known as acropachy or clubbing. It is also noticed that fingernail growth increases but, in some, the nail becomes soft and tears off easily. It was further noticed that an alarming condition develops in some patients known as onycholysis, a condition where the upper edge of the fingernails becomes partially separated from the fingertip.

Symptoms of thyrotoxicosis

- Weight loss despite an increased appetite
- Increased or, in some people, decreased appetite
- Irritability
- Weakness and fatigue
- Diarrhoea or, in some people, constipation
- Sweating
- Tremor
- Mental illness, which may vary from anxiety to psychosis
- Heat intolerance
- Loss of libido
- Reduced menstruation or complete absence (oligmenorrhoea or amenorrhoea)

How is thyrotoxicosis diagnosed?

Your General Practitioner will normally conduct a blood test called the thyroid function test. A blood sample will be taken by a trained person, either your practice nurse or in the nearest hospital, or even your own GP if it is urgent. During this examination, the blood test is used to evaluate the function of the thyroid gland and may include the measurements of the hormone that regulates the function of the thyroid gland, as well as direct measurements of the different forms of the thyroid hormone produced and secreted by the thyroid gland.

Thyroid ultrasound (USS) or thyroid uptake scans may also be necessary to locate hot (over activity) and cold (no activity) spots.

What causes thyrotoxicosis?

There are four main causes of thyrotoxicosis:

- A generalised enlargement of the thyroid (Graves' disease)
- An overactive solitary lump in the thyroid (Plummer's disease)
- Overactivity in a multinodular goitre (Toxic multinodular goitre)
- Inflammation of the thyroid resulting in release of excess thyroid hormone (Thyroiditis)

Less common causes of thyrotoxicosis

There are also some less common causes of thyrotoxicosis, such as:

Intake of excess thyroid hormone (Thyrotoxicosis Facticia) or iodine containing agents, e.g., amiodarone or contrast agents

- Congenital thyrotoxicosis (inherited from the mother) or family history
- Transient thyrotoxicosis (occurs in twenty per cent women with previous thyrotoxicosis)
- Normal thyroid function during pregnancy (Post-partum thyroiditis)
- Thyroid "storm", which is rarely seen and it is brought by physical or surgical stress that causes a massive release of the thyroid hormone into the bloodstream (Thyroid Crisis)
- Ectopic tumour that produces excessive amounts of THS which causes overactivity of the thyroid (Ectopic Hyperthyroidism)

Hyperthyroidism

Hyperthyroidism or overactive thyroid is a common cause of thyrotoxicosis, meaning that the thyroid gland becomes overactive and produces plenty of hormones over the normal limit. A person will then become thyrotoxic, a condition known as thyrotoxicosis.

Causes of hyperthyroidism (overactive thyroid)

The common cause of hyperthyroidism is Graves' disease, which is responsible for about 80 per cent of the cases. Graves' disease is an autoimmune thyroid disease and is the next common autoimmune thyroid disease after Hashimoto's Thyroiditis. Graves' disease is named after Robert James Graves, a physician of the nineteenth century who published a description of three patients who suffered from this condition in 1835 in the London Medical and Surgical Journal. Graves' disease affects men, women and children from all races across the globe, including the rich and the poor. It was noticed that it affects women more, usually between the ages of twenty and forty.

How does Graves' disease work?

Graves' disease is a condition in which an abnormal antibody called thyroid-stimulating antibody (TSA) or thyroid-stimulating immunoglobulin (TSI) is produced. The TSA then stimulates the thyroid gland into vastly overproducing the thyroid hormone, which is normally controlled by the pituitary gland. The thyroid triggers are tricked and stimulated by these abnormal antibodies. The result of this activity is called hyperthyroidism, which in turn will present the symptoms of thyrotoxicosis with a small goitre at times. But, this is not easy to palpate during medical examination.

Symptoms of Graves' disease

The symptoms of Graves' disease are the same as that of thyrotoxicosis. However, there are a few additional complications unique to Graves' disease, such as:

- Thyroid Eye Disease (TED). TED or Graves' ophthalmopathy (GO) or Graves' orbitopathy can be quite severe in people affected by Graves' disease. It has been reported that the majority of thyrotoxic Graves' disease patients suffer from measurable TED.
- Heart disease. Graves' disease can also worsen or lead to heart disease in patients who are thyrotoxic due to the excessive amount of thyroid hormone in the body
- Diabetes. If a person is thyrotoxic, the metabolism increases. Thus, a person develops an increased need for insulin especially in type 1 or in type 2 diabetes, which can put a patient in a high risk category.
- Loss of pigmentation (vitiligo). This is an autoimmune condition commonly found in people with Graves' disease. It is a condition

that attacks the melanin, which contains the skin cells. It also causes the development of thick skin over the lower legs called pretibial myxedema. This means the skin becomes firm, swollen and darker in the affected areas. It is thought to be a reaction to the autoimmune antibody of Graves' disease. This condition is normally treated with steroid creams or ointments. In some people, the fingernails become remarkably thick causing the ends of the fingers to thicken. It also causes loss of hair which can be permanent.

The diagnosis of Graves' disease

The signs of Graves' disease are in many patients obvious. They might develop goitre with the usual signs of thyrotoxicosis. In some cases, patients only present the symptoms of TED, which is a common sign of Graves' disease. If the signs are already there, a doctor only has to confirm the diagnosis with a blood test that checks the thyroid hormone levels and the presence of anti-thyroid antibodies. Therefore, if you suspect that you might have Graves' disease, please get it checked out by your GP as this can have serious consequences.

Treatment of Graves' disease

Treating the roots of Graves' disease is difficult because it involves the treatment of hyperthyroidism. However, various treatments are suitable for Graves' disease with advantages and disadvantages. In order to treat hyperthyroidism, the thyroid gland is either destroyed completely or just a piece of it is removed. These procedures are called total thyroidectomy if the whole thyroid is removed, or partial thyroidectomy if it is just a piece no matter how small. It can also be treated with radioactive iodine. The reason for both these treatments is to make the patient deliberately hypothyroid, meaning the person goes from overactive to underactive and then he or she will be put on thyroid hormone treatment for life.

The main reason for both these treatments is really to speed up the process so that the person does not suffer for too long with the illness. The Graves' disease will normally cause the thyroid gland to burn out, but a person can be treated with antithyroid medication that can be stopped once the thyroid has returned to normal levels. It is also important for people to know that the overall goal of the treatments is to bring the patients to a hypothyroid level and to start on a thyroid hormone called thyroxine for life.

Antithyroid medication

Two common medications are used to treat Graves' disease, namely Propylthiouracil (PTU) and Carbimazole (Tapazole). These drugs prevent the thyroid gland from manufacturing thyroid hormone and are usually a way of managing the Graves' disease in the short term. The drugs are useful in specific circumstances such as:

- Severe thyrotoxicosis, in order to lower the thyroid hormone levels before radioactive treatment
- Graves' disease during pregnancy
- Severe TED in patients who are reluctant to undergo thyroid surgery
- Mild thyrotoxicosis in Graves' disease with a very small goitre
- Thyrotoxicosis in any patient in an unstable clinical condition or in a thyroid storm
- Patients who have strong fears about radioactive iodine

Autonomous Toxic Nodules (ATNs)

Autonomous toxic nodules (ATNs), also known as toxic adenomas or autonomous toxic thyroid nodules, are single thyroid nodules that independently make too much thyroid hormone without the need for TSH to stimulate them ATNs are suspected if a person becomes thyrotoxic, their TSH level is low, and there is a lump on the thyroid gland.

The thyroid toxic nodule is normally diagnosed with a radioactive iodine thyroid scan.

Toxic multinodular goitre

In some people, the thyroid glands form multiple nodules that can be usually felt during physical examination of the thyroid. These nodules start to produce too much thyroid hormone and do not require TSH to do so. In this situation, a radioactive iodine thyroid scan will show the toxic nodules, whether multiple or single. It is normally called toxic nodule or toxic multinodular goitre, if any.

Thyroid hormone overdose

Thyroid hormone overdose becomes a cause of thyrotoxicosis if the thyroid hormone is given without ground base on the appropriate monitoring after using appropriate laboratory tests. The other reason is if the person is not compliant with the treatment. This can happen because of complications arising from the illness such as memory loss. For instance, they may forget that they have taken their thyroid hormone pill and might take another dose. On the other hand, there are people who mistakenly believe that taking excessive thyroid hormone doses by purpose will help relieve the symptoms of fatigue or lack of energy. The opposite is, in fact, true. Thyrotoxicosis can also occur in patients who are on a high dose of thyroid hormone to suppress the TSH, for instance in thyroid cancer patients. If the dosage is poorly adjusted, it leads to thyrotoxicosis.

Misuse of thyroid hormone

The misuse of the thyroid hormone was common between the 1950s and the 1970s. Levothyroxine Sodium was prescribed to overweight or obese women, and they were told it would speed up their metabolism, which would result in the desired weight loss.

Thyroiditis

Thyroiditis is the inflammation of the thyroid gland, which may cause thyrotoxicosis. This means that the thyroid gland swells in many cases due to viral infection. However, rare cases of bacterial infection have been found that might need urgent hospitalisation and intravenous antibodies (IVA).

Types of thyroiditis

Subacute viral thyroiditis

There are various types of thyroiditis, such as subacute viral thyroiditis causes pain in the neck. This type of thyroiditis is also known as de Quervain's. Thyroiditis is named after the Swiss physician who first described the infection. This infection seems to be common in North America although Hashimoto's disease tends to be forty times more common. This infection occurs more in women. This type of thyroiditis usually triggers the flu. Its symptoms are: tiredness, muscular aches and pains, headache and fever, and swelling of the thyroid gland as the illness progresses, which makes the thyroid gland very tender and sore. It becomes hurtful when swallowing, it feels like stabbing in the neck and one might become thyrotoxic.

The treatment for this is to take aspirin, which alleviates the swelling and inflammation. If there is thyrotoxicosis in severe form, beta-blockers may be prescribed to slow the heart rate or cortisone analogs are given normal prednisone.

Silent thyroiditis

This form of thyroiditis is given its name because it is a very tricky infection and difficult to diagnose until the symptoms become severe. However, it is debatable whether this is a unique thyroiditis or a type of Hashimoto's Thyroiditis that is not associated with goitre. This is because most forms of autoimmune thyroiditis, with lymphocytes invading the thyroid gland, are commonly called Hashimoto's Thyroiditis. The only difference between the two types of thyroiditis is that a silent thyroiditis runs a painless course but is the same as subacute viral thyroiditis and Hashitoxicosis.

Post-partum thyroiditis

The name post-partum thyroiditis is a general label referring to silent thyroiditis after delivery. This normally causes mild hyperthyroidism and short-lived Hashimoto's type of thyroiditis that causes mild hypothyroidism. Post-partum thyroid peroxidase (TPO) antibodies are more likely to experience post-partum thyroiditis.

Acute suppurative thyroiditis

This is also known as acute bacterial thyroiditis, which is a very rare condition. The term suppurative refers to the presence of bacteria and pus which is common in the thyroid gland. This means that the thyroid gland has suffered a dramatic pus-forming bacterial infection similar to the ones that cause boils and abscesses.

Riedel's thyroiditis

This type of thyroiditis is the rarest. It is a condition where the thyroid gland is infiltrated by scar tissue through the gland, which binds it to the surrounding portions of the neck. This makes the thyroid very tender and hard like wood. Because of this, the attachment of the gland to other parts of the body, the windpipe for example, will feel restricted. The vocal cord will also be affected, making it difficult to swallow. Riedel's Thyroiditis is normally diagnosed through a biopsy in order to rule out cancer, because the cause of this condition is still unknown. The only treatment for this condition is surgical removal of the front part of the gland and sending it for histological investigation by a pathologist/ histologist who has expertise in thyroid problems.

Thyroid nodules

The word nodule in the thyroid context means a lump. In most cases, thyroid nodules that are cancerous are first found as nodules in the thyroid gland, or as a lump or enlarged lymph node in other places of the neck. Many of these nodes are benign, meaning they are not cancerous. However, most of these nodules are colliding nodules which do not produce too much thyroid hormone. Thyroid nodules sometimes also come in the form of a cyst which can be partially cystic (fluid base) and partially solid. Most of these cysts are also said to be benign but some might contain thyroid cancer in their wall.

Thyroid cancer

Thyroid cancer has the same percentage of prevalence as any other illness, two per cent in men and women of all ages, and four per cent in children.

Causes of thyroid cancer

No definite cause of thyroid cancer has yet been identified. It has, however, been noticed that people who are most at risk of thyroid cancer are those who were exposed to radiation or RAI from a nuclear fallout. This means that when a healthy thyroid gland is exposed to RAI, its cells can develop breaks in their chromosomes. This can lead to cancer.

Types of thyroid cancers

There are common and uncommon thyroid cancers.

Common thyroid cancers

- Papillary thyroid cancer. This is a frightening form of thyroid cancer because it tends to spread to the lymph nodes in the neck. It accounts for about eighty per cent of all thyroid cancers.
- Tall cell papillary cancer. Tall cell papillary cancer spreads rapidly and has a greater chance of losing the ability of sucking up the iodine during treatment. Therefore, it is likely to recur.

- Follicular thyroid cancer. Follicular cancers occur three times more in women. It affects more people in the forty to sixty age group and make up about ten per cent of thyroid cancers. It is found to be less aggressive in people under forty because it responds better to RAI in younger people. It is also believed that fifteen per cent of follicular cancers spread to the lymph nodes.
- Hurtble cell cancer. This type of cancer is also called oncocytic thyroid cancer. It is a type of a follicular cancer though it is less common than follicular cancer and accounts for up to four per cent of all thyroid cancers. It is more common in people in their midfifties or older, and does not tend to spread to the lymph nodes unlike follicular cancer.

Uncommon thyroid cancers

- Medullary thyroid cancer. This type of cancer is rare and can be spontaneous or inherited (FMTC). It involves the parafollicular cell (C cell), which does not produce thyroid hormone or take up iodine. Therefore, using RAI as treatment is pointless. The best way to treat this type of cancer is through prevention.
- Unresponsive aggressive thyroid cancer tumours. This cancer and anaplastic thyroid cancer are undifferentiated. Follicular or papillary thyroid cancers may turn into anaplastic, which is an aggressive and untreatable form of thyroid cancer.

Treatment for thyroid cancers

Most thyroid cancers, especially the papillary and follicular thyroid cancers, are treated either surgically or with RAI. During the surgical procedure, the thyroid gland is either removed completely or partially, or sometimes just a lob. It depends on the severity. If only one lob is removed, it is called lobectomy; if a tiny bit of the thyroid gland is removed, it is called partial thyroidectomy; and where the whole thyroid gland has been removed, it is called total thyroidectomy. A neck dissection is when some of the lymph nodes in the neck that might have had cancer have also been removed.

RAI

The effectiveness of RAI depends on the type of cancer and the stage of advancement of the disease. For example, if it is an aggressive one such as follicular or tall cell papillary cancer, then the person affected needs radioactive iodine, either in capsule or in liquid form, as these two forms are the only ones that will be easily taken up by the thyroid gland. It will then kill them. (See under the subhead, Treatment of thyrotoxicosis.)

Hormone therapy

After the thyroid gland has been surgically removed or destroyed with the RAI, a person normally goes hypo or underactive. Therefore, the person will then need thyroid hormone medication for life so that it helps him or her with the body metabolism. They will also need a TSH suppressive dosage.

Beta-blockers

If the symptoms of thyrotoxicosis persist, you need a dose of beta-blockers to slow the heart rate.

Treatments

The person affected will normally be referred to a specialist for treatments, which might include:

Drug treatment

Drug treatment normally includes carbimazole or propylthiouracil, depending on the individual. Beta-blockers might also be prescribed to slow the heart rate.

Radioiodine

This has increasingly become the first line of treatment, especially in teenagers and older patients. It is given as 200-600MBq, and some people might need a second dose of radioiodine normally given as a drink. On entering the body, it is taken up by the thyroid gland, which leads to destruction of the gland.

Advantages: It is an inexpensive and definitive method of treating thyrotoxicosis.

Disadvantages: It cannot be given to pregnant women or breastfeeding mothers. Women must be advised not to get pregnant for at least four months after radioactive iodine treatment has been given.

- Radioactive iodine may also worsen eye disease in Graves' thyrotoxicosis
- Patient has to be informed that radioactive iodine is cleared via the urine and can thus be passed on
- There is no close contact with children and pregnant women even if they are members of your own household. Patients are also required to sleep separately for a week after the administration of radioactive iodine.
- Under-thyroid gland functioning (hypothyroidism) is a potential and common complication. In fifty to eighty per cent cases, patients who have this treatment need a long-term follow up of thyroid function tests.

Surgery

If surgical intervention is needed, the surgeons will decide on the removal of the whole thyroid gland, or a part of it.

Complications: Common complications after surgery are bleeding, under-parathyroidism, and vocal cord paralysis. Therefore, patients need follow up over a number of years as they may develop hypothyroidism.

For more information about thyrotoxicosis, please contact the British or any country's thyroid Foundation.

Coping with Thyrotoxicosis, Heart Failure, and Hypertension

Thyrotoxicosis and hyperthyroidism

Overview

Many people, including doctors, nurses and thyroid patients are confused between the two terms hyperthyroidism, which means an overactive gland, and thyrotoxicosis, which means too much thyroid hormone. Thus, one can say hyperthyroidism and thyrotoxicosis are cousins that often pass as twins. This means that an overactive thyroid gland (hyperthyroid) produces too much thyroid hormone, which results in thyrotoxicosis and its symptoms. However, thyrotoxicosis, or too much thyroid hormone, can also be caused by other thyroid diseases, commonly the Graves' disease and also by taking too much or a high dose of thyroid hormone as medication.

How does your thyroid gland work?

The thyroid gland is often referred to as a butterfly-shaped gland, but it is also shaped like the capital letter H. Each side of the H or butterfly is called a lobe while the centre or the body of the butterfly is called the isthmus. The thyroid gland is located in the lower part of your neck in front of your windpipe and is basically wrapped around the windpipe. We can say the butterfly hugs the windpipe.

What is thyrotoxicosis?

Thyrotoxicosis occurs when there is an increased level of the thyroid hormone in a person's blood. Thyrotoxicosis affects two per cent of the population of the United Kingdom and is ten times more common in females. In forty per cent patients, the disease is self-limiting.

How many people are affected and who is mostly affected?

According to the Department of Health in England, the following are recorded as hospital statistics (2002-03):

- 00.027% (3,382) of hospital consultant episodes were for thyrotoxicosis
- 22% of hospital consultant episodes for thyrotoxicosis were for men
- 78% of hospital consultant episodes for thyrotoxicosis were for women
- 87% of hospital consultant episodes for thyrotoxicosis required hospital admission
- 32% of hospital consultant episodes for thyrotoxicosis required emergency hospital admission
- 64% of hospital consultant episodes for thyrotoxicosis occurred in patients 15-59 years old
- 15% of hospital consultant episodes for thyrotoxicosis occurred in people over 75 years of age.
- 6.5 days was the average length of stay in hospital due to thyrotoxicosis
- 16% of hospital consultant episodes for thyrotoxicosis were single-day episodes

In Caucasians, thyrotoxicosis affects 2%-3% of women and 0.2%-0.3% of men. Thyrotoxicosis affects more women than men with a ratio of 9:1, and has been reported at 0.8 per 1,000 per year in women and 0.1 in men during the same follow-up period.

What are the signs of thyrotoxicosis?

There are many signs of thyrotoxicosis, but the following are the prominent ones.

- Sweaty and warm palms
- Fine tremor
- Fast heartbeat (called "tachycardia"), which might be with or without atrial fibrillation—common in elderly people
- Hair thinning or diffuse alopecia
- Brisk reflexes
- Goitre prominent in neck
- Muscle weakness, sometimes wasting

Other symptoms of thyrotoxicosis include the following:

- Weight loss despite an increased appetite
- Increased—or in some people decreased—appetite
- Irritability
- Weakness and fatigue
- Diarrhoea or, in some, constipation
- Mental illness, which may vary from anxiety to psychosis
- Heat intolerance
- Loss of libido
- Reduction in menstruation or complete absence (oligomenorrhea or amenorrhea)

How is thyrotoxicosis diagnosed?

A general practitioner will normally conduct a blood test called the thyroid function test. During this examination, the blood test is used to evaluate the function of the thyroid gland. It may include the measurements of the hormone that regulates the function of the thyroid gland as well as direct measurements of the different forms of the thyroid hormone produced and secreted by the thyroid gland.

The following investigations may also be necessary.

- Thyroid ultrasound

- Thyroid uptake scans to locate hot (overactivity) and cold (no activity) spots

What causes thyrotoxicosis?

The following are the main causes of thyrotoxicosis.

- A generalised enlargement of the thyroid (Graves' disease)
- An overactive solitary lump in the thyroid (Plummer's disease)
- Overactivity in a multinodular goitre (Toxic multinodular goitre)
- Inflammation of the thyroid resulting in release of excess thyroid hormone (thyroiditis)
- Intake of excess thyroid hormone (thyrotoxicosis factitia) or iodine containing agents (e.g., amiodarone or contrast agents)
- Congenital thyrotoxicosis inherited from mother's family
- Transient thyrotoxicosis, which occurs in 20 per cent women who had previous thyrotoxicosis, and normal thyroid function during pregnancy (post-partum thyroiditis)
- A thyroid "storm" or thyroid crisis (rarely seen; brought on by physical or surgical stress that causes a massive release of the thyroid hormone into the bloodstream)
- An ectopic tumour that produces excessive amounts of TSH and causes overactivity of the thyroid (ectopic hyperthyroidism)

How is thyrotoxicosis treated?

The person affected will be normally referred to a specialist for treatments, which might include the following.

Drug treatment. The common drugs used include carbimazole or propylthiouracil, depending on the individual. Beta-blockers may also be prescribed to slow down a high heart rate, if present.

Radioiodine. This has increasingly become the first line of treatment, especially in teenagers and older patients. It is normally given in a capsule form to be taken orally. On entering the body, it is taken up by the thyroid gland, which leads to the destruction of the gland.

Surgery. If a surgical intervention is needed, the surgeons will decide whether to remove the whole thyroid gland or just part of it. Common complications following surgery include bleeding, hypoparathyroidism, and vocal cord paralysis. Therefore, patients need follow-up over a number of years as they may develop hypothyroidism.

Heart Failure

What is heart failure?

Heart failure is a serious medical condition in which the heart does not pump blood around the body as well as it should. This means that the blood can't deliver enough oxygen and nourishment to the body to allow it to work normally. This may cause muscle fatigue. It also means that the body can't eliminate waste products properly, which leads to a buildup of fluid in the lungs and other parts of the body, such as the legs and abdomen.

How does heart failure develop?

A heart failure often develops because a person has or had a medical condition such as a coronary artery disease, a heart attack, or high blood pressure, which has damaged or put extra workload on the heart.

People of any age can develop heart failure, but clearly it becomes more common with increasing age. It has been noted that 1% of people under the age of 65 have heart failure, and seven per cent of people of 75-84 years age; this increases to 15 per cent in people older than 85 years. It has also been noted that heart failure is the most common cause of hospital admissions in patients over 65 years of age. However, although it is called heart failure this does not mean the heart is about to stop working, but only means that the heart is having difficulties in meeting the needs of the body.

What are the causes of heart failure?

Some contributing factors to heart failure are stroke, smoking, overweight, eating foods containing too much fat and cholesterol, and physical inactivity. Apart from the contributing factors, there are also medical conditions that can lead to heart failure if not controlled soon. Such as the following:

- Coronary artery disease
- Past heart attack (myocardial infarction)
- High blood pressure (hypertension)
- Heart muscle disease (dilated cardiomyopathy, hypertrophic cardiomyopathy) or inflammation (myocarditis)
- Heart defects present at birth (congenital heart diseases)

- Severe lung disease
- Diabetes
- Other conditions (low red blood cell count, called anemia; overactive thyroid which causes thyrotoxicosis; abnormal heart rhythm, called arrhythmia or dysrhythmia).

What are the signs and symptoms of heart failure?

The common symptoms of a heart failure include breathlessness, tiredness, and swollen feet and ankles. Other symptoms depend on which side of the heart is most affected.

How is heart failure diagnosed?

A GP will ask the patient about symptoms and examine the patient; he or she might also ask for the medical history. In addition to these the GP may order blood and urine tests and other tests to check blood count, liver function, and markers of heart failure like:

- Electrocardiogram (ECG)—a test that measures the electrical activity of the heart to see how well it is working
- Echocardiogram (heart ultrasound scan) to show the pumping action of the heart and valves
- Chest x-ray (to rule out other conditions)

What are the complications of heart failure?

People with heart failure are at risk of the following:

- Poor quality of life due to difficulty in carrying out everyday activities
- Depression (a third of people with heart failure develop severe depression)
- Irregular heart beat (arrhythmia), which can be fatal
- Damage to the brain caused by blood clots (stroke)
- Bloods clots in the lungs or legs
- Liver congestion

How is heart failure treated?

ACE inhibitors. A range of medication can be given, such as a group of inhibitors that help the heart to pump more blood. These are often used to lower blood pressure. They are generally recommended for all patients with heart failure.

Beta-blockers. Beta-blockers are commonly used for treating high blood pressure, and studies have shown that specific ones can improve the life expectancy in some patients with heart failure

Diuretics. Diuretics are a type of medication commonly known as water tablets and are the most used in patients with heart failure. They help in reducing the amount of fluids in the human body by making a person urinate more often. This should help one breathe more easily by removing fluids in the lungs and be more active by reducing leg swelling.

Anticoagulants. Blood clots are more likely to form in people with heart failure. These can be carried in the circulation and may block narrow vessels, preventing blood from reaching some areas of the body. If this happens in the brain, it is called a stroke. Therefore, anticoagulants or blood thinners are used to thin the blood.

Other Treatment

Pacemaker: A pacemaker is a small device, usually implanted under the skin in the upper chest. Electrical signals are sent from the pacemaker to the heart to stimulate it to beat at a specific rate. Pacemakers are usually fitted under local anesthetic; this completely blocks the feeling in the chest and the patient remains awake during an operation. If a person has severe heart failure (an ECG appearance called "left bundle branch block"), a special type of pacemaker called a resynchronisation (biventricular) pacemaker can be helpful.

Implantable cardioverter-defibrillator (ICD): An ICD is similar to a pacemaker. However, an ICD can monitor heart rhythm and deliver a small electric shock to return a heartbeat to normal if it detects a problem. As with pacemakers, ICDs are usually fitted under local anaesthetic.

Transplantation: For some people who have severe heart failure, a heart transplant may be an option. This can be a very successful procedure, although complications such as rejection of the donor heart can occur. Transplantation is limited by the number of donor hearts available.

How can heart failure be prevented?

A heart-healthy lifestyle can reduce risk of heart failure by reducing the risk of coronary artery disease and high blood pressure. Maintaining a healthy weight, not smoking, being physically active most days, and eating a balanced diet are all recommended to prevent heart conditions. It is also sensible to stick to moderate drinking and to keep a check on one's blood pressure and cholesterol level.

High Blood Pressure (Hypertension)

As many as one in five is believed to be suffering from high blood pressure, medically known as hypertension. This is a situation were the blood is forced through the human body under constant high pressure. Hypertension is diagnosed when the systolic pressure is consistently greater than 140mmHg and the diastolic more than 90mmHg.

What is high blood pressure and how does it exist?

Blood pressure exists because a person's heart pumps bloods around his or her body, which is a closed system and not like a boiler pumping water through a series of central heating pipes. The pressure in your arteries therefore depends on a number of factors, including the volume of fluids inside your circulation, how hard your heart is pumping at any given time, and the elasticity or resistance of the vessels the blood is passing through. Normal blood pressure varies naturally through the day and night, going up and down depending on one's emotions and the level of activities a person is involved in. If a person has high blood pressure, it will remain considerably high even during sleep.

The heart alternately contracts and relaxes as it pumps to produce the heartbeat. Each contraction produces a surge in pressure. The highest pressure reached in the arteries during this surge is known as the systolic pressure as it is due to contraction (systole) of the heart. As the heart rest between the beats, the blood pressure falls and the lowest blood pressure recorded while the heart rests (diastole) is called the diastolic pressure.

How is blood pressure measured?

Blood pressure is measured by using a specific masjien called a sphygmomanometer. This instrument is normally put around a person's arm; the cuff that goes around the arm is inflatable with a small pump to push air into the cuff and to push a column of mercury to record the pressure within the cuff.

Hypertension and its diagnoses

Hypertension, or high blood pressure, means that the blood is forced through a person's system under constant high pressure. It is diagnosed when the systolic pressure is consistently greater than 140mmHg and the diastolic pressure consistently greater than 90mmHg. A systolic blood pressure between 140-160mmHg and a diastolic of 90-95mmHg is sometimes referred to as mild hypertension.

In people with hypertension, the body systems for correcting high or low blood pressure don't seem to work properly. Therefore, blood pressure is maintained at an elevated level compared to normal. However, the condition can be reversed once diet and lifestyle changes with necessary anti-hypertensive drugs have been introduced after the diagnosis has been made.

Symptoms

It is an unfortunate that people with blood pressure notice very little of the symptoms of blood pressure. The only symptom they might notice is a pounding sensation in their ears or a splitting headache. This has resulted in hypertension becoming a silent killer as it usually creeps up on a person without a warning. Some people will still feel well even if the blood pressure is very high, and manage to continue with normal duties unless it really goes through the roof.

Types of hypertension

Around 90% of people who suffer from high blood pressure have no obvious single cause and are said to have primary or essential hypertension. The remaining one in ten has underlying problems or causes such as kidney, hormonal problems or drug-related side effects, and are said to have secondary hypertension.

There is also another type of hypertension called the malignant hypertension. This is the most dangerous hypertension, which can damage a person's internal organs in a very short time.

Causes of hypertension

There are various factors that contribute to the cause of hypertension such as, inheritance, this means that high blood pressure runs in some families; or developmental and environmental factors such as diet and lifestyle, which can be addressed either by the individuals themselves or through health education.

Treatment of high blood pressure

High blood pressure is normally treated with medications called anti-hypertensive drugs, whose main aim is to bring the diastolic blood pressure below 85mmHg or the systolic below 140mmHg. There are six main groups of medications which are used to treat high blood pressure, such as:

Thiazide diuretics. These are the first-line treatment in the elderly and can sometimes be combined with another anti-hypertensive drug from other groups such as a beta-blocker or ACE inhibitors. An example of thiazide diuretics is bendrofluazide.

Beta-blockers. Beta-blockers are thought to lower the blood pressure through a combination of actions such as:

- Altering the way the nerve signals cause some blood vessels to dilate or constrict
- Slowing down the heart rate to 60 beats per minute
- Reducing the force of contraction of the heart
- Decreasing the workload of the heart and cardiac output
- Lowering the secretion of the kidney hormone called renin
- Reducing sensitivity of the blood pressure sensors (baroreceptors)
- Blocking the stress hormone or adrenaline receptors
- Having an effect on the brain

In general beta-blockers are also thought to be used as a first line of treatment in young people with hypertension and people who have coronary heart diseases.

Alpha-blockers. They lower blood pressure by dilating both arteries and veins. Examples of these are doxazosin, indoramin and terazosin to mention just a few. They are more useful in older males who suffer from both high blood pressure and noncancerous enlarged prostate gland.

Calcium channel blockers. They help lower blood pressure by:

- Blocking the transportation of calcium ions through the cell membranes
- Relaxing the muscles in the arterial walls and reducing their spasm
- Dilating the peripheral veins to encourage pooling of blood
- Reducing the force of contraction of the heart

Examples of this group of medication are diltiazem, felodipine, isradipine, and nifidipine.

ACE inhibitors. They lower blood pressure by preventing the formation of a substance called angiotensin II, a very powerful constrictor of both blood vessels. ACE inhibitors dilate both small arteries and veins. They are also thought to increase the flow of blood to the kidneys.

Angiotensin II Antagonists. They are similar to ACE inhibitors. Although they don't actually inhibit the angiotensin-converting enzyme, they block it from producing similar effects. Some of these medications are losartan and valsartan.

General Coping Strategies for Both Conditions

Relaxation and regular exercise may help in dealing with the pain people often suffer from both these conditions. It is also advisable to keep an eye on what one eats, such as reducing salt, alcohol, etc. If the person is depressed, then the GP might refer him or her to a counselor for further management. People with thyrotoxicosis and heart failure are also advised to join local available thyrotoxicosis and heart failure self-help groups. The following are also recommended where applicable: losing weight, cutting down on alcohol, and stress management.

Finally, complementary therapies might also be helpful. These include acupuncture, aromatherapy, Bach Flower Remedies, biochemical tissue salts, chiropractics, healing herbalism, homoeopathy, meditation, osteopathy, reflexology, shiatsu, and visualisation.

For more information on both conditions, please contact the British Thyroid Foundation, the British Hypertension Society, and The British Heart Foundation as well as any other source of information around the world.

ABOUT THE AUTHOR

Mrs. Hedwig Taaru qualified as a general registered nurse at the Oshakati Nursing College in Namibia in 1980, and specialised in midwifery in 1981 at the Onandjokwe Nursing College. Mrs. Taaru then worked as a general nurse in adult medicine in the Oshakati Hospital. She furthered her study at the Windhoek Training College in primary health care and provision of family planning. Mrs. Taaru worked at the Old Niek Clinic as a qualified nurse, providing preventative and curative care to the community in the area and beyond.

She had worked as a primary health care district supervisor in Oshikuku district, where she trained heath care assistants in the same hospital and also worked as a general nurse.

Mrs. Taaru was later transferred back to the regional directorate, where she performed various functions ranging including training officers for the local community-based program, information communication, and as a maternal and child health program officer. She determined to further her study in 1996-1997 at the University of London, where she subsequently completed her master of science in maternal and child health care. Returning to Namibia, she continued in the same roles as before. Mrs. Taaru dedicated herself to these functions until 2000, when she decided to leave the country and applied for a nursing position in the United Kingdom. She was accepted in a department of trauma and orthopedics, where she earned the trust of her colleagues as a dedicated nurse. At one point, she received the following comment, "You are a saint, life saver, and a good nurse. You don't deserve to be a 'D' grade." Mrs. Taaru applied the knowledge she had acquired over the years. In 2004, she applied for postgraduate study in heath and medical science through a health care trust at the University of Reading in the UK. She only managed to study for the first three years, at which time her illness started to become unbearable and she could no longer cope with the combined stress of work, study, and illness. She decided to give up her study. At that time, she did not know what was really going on; she only knew she had high blood pressure and at one point was diagnosed with a heart murmur, which was cleared up—only God knows how—with no medical intervention. After she did not receive approval of her first request to transfer from postgraduate to PhD/MPH studies, she decided to write to her supervisor suggesting that she continue her studies through distance learning. She continued to work as a nurse at the local hospital, although she was on and off work. In October 2007, she dropped her studies. Although the illness had started to reach its peak in March–April, she had always denied that she was ill because she could not put a finger on anything apart from the two above-mentioned conditions and weight loss. She sometimes told her colleagues, who asked her about her weight loss, that she was on a diet. In December 2007, Mrs. Taaru was diagnosed with thyrotoxicosis with multinodular goitre, heart failure, and hypertension. She battled these three facets of her illness until 2009, when she realised that she could no longer be a nurse and a patient at the same time. As things were going very slowly and the condition had become frightening, she decided to put in her resignation instead of going on ill health retirement. Mrs. Taaru resigned from the trust in January 2009 and, having made a good recovery, she is considering volunteer work, completing her study, and performing charity work to keep busy while recovering.

APPENDIX 1

Thyroid Resources

American Thyroid Association, www.thyroid.org

Thyroid Foundation of Canada, www.thyroid.ca

European Thyroid Association, www.eurothyroid.com

Latin America Thyroid Society, www.lats.org

Australian Thyroid Foundation, www.thyroidfoundation.com.au

Thyroid Foundation of Brazil, email: *medneto@uol.com.br*

Denmark: Thyreoidea Landsforeningen, www.thyreoidea.dk

Thyroid Foundation of Finland, *www.kolombus.fi/kilpirauhasliitto*

L'Association Francaise des Malades de la Thyroide, *www.thyro-asso.org*

Schilddrusen Liga Deutschland e.V. (SLD), www.schilddruesenliga.de

Associazione Italiana Basedowiani e Tiroidei. email: *emma99@libero.it*

Thyroid Foundation of Japan, *www.hata.ne.jp/tfj/*

Schildklierstichting Nederland, *www.schildklier.nl*

Norway: Norsk Thyreoideaforbund, *www.stoffskifte.org*

Georgian Union of Diabetes and Endocrine Associations, email: *diabet@access.sanet.ge*

Skoldkortelforening I Stockholm, www.skoldkortelforeningen.se

British Thyroid Foundation, www.btf-thyroid.org

APPENDIX 2

Definitions and Terms

Acute suppurative thyroiditis, A very rare form of bacterial thyroiditis.in which pus and inflammation occur. It is normally treated with antibiotics.

Adam's apple. The thyroid cartilage.

Amiodarone. Amiodarone is a medication used to treat heart rhythm abnormalities. It is well known in for causing different types of thyroid problems.

Anaplastic thyroid cancer. A very rare and very aggressive hard to treat thyroid cancer with poor outcomes. It accounts for about 1.6 per cent of all thyroid cancers.

Angina. A chest pain due to blockage of blood supply to the heart muscle.

Antithyroid medication. Drugs that are used to treat Graves' diseases, thyrotoxicosis and other thyroid problems, which cause too much formation of the thyroid hormone. The common ones are propylthiouracil (PTU) and carbimazole.

Apathetic hyperthyroidism. Hyperthyroidism without clear symptoms of thyrotoxicosis. It is usually diagnosed in patients over sixty.

Arrhythmia. Abnormal heart rhythm.

Atherosclerotic cardiovascular disease (ASCVD). A condition referred to as a fatty blockage of a blood vessel anywhere in the body that can put a person at risk of heart attack or even a stroke.

Atrial fibrillation. A disordered rapid irregular heart rhythm.

Autoimmune thyroid disease. A thyroid disorder where the thyroid antibodies are attacking the thyroid gland as in Hashimoto's Thyroiditis or Graves' disease.

Autonomous toxic nodules (ATNs). Lumps that are making thyroid hormones on their own and do not respond to TSH. This can be a single nodule or multinodular nodules.

Benign. A noncancerous condition.

Beta-blockers. A type of medication that is used to block adrenaline and slow the heart rate. It is commonly used in people with thyrotoxicosis.

Bradycardia. A slow heartbeat which is common in patients with hypothyroidism

Catecholamines. Referred to adrenalines and related hormones.

Congenital hypothyroidism. Underactive thyroid that is present from birth.

Congestive heart failure. A condition where the heart is unable to pump blood to the whole body.

Cyst. A fluid-filled lump, which is usually noncancerous

Differentiated thyroid cancer cells. Cancer cells that function like normal thyroid follicular cells.

Euthyroid. A normal thyroid function.

Exophthalmometer. An instrument that measures the degree to which the eyes protrude from the skull. It is used in people with bulging watery eyes, which is a symptom of thyroid eye disease (exophthalmos).

Follicular thyroid cancer. A type of thyroid cancer that is usually treatable, either by surgery or RAI, and normally with good effect. This type of cancer accounts for roughly ten per cent of all thyroid cancers.

Free T4. The portion of all the T4 that is able to be taken up into each body cell and do the job of an effective thyroid hormone.

Free T4 test. An appropriate blood test to measure the free T4 levels.

Generalised anxiety disorders (GAD). A condition called a psychiatric or psychological disorder in which one suffers from persistent worry and anxiety without any relief even if there is a good reason not to worry.

Gestational hyperthyroidism (overactive thyroid). An overactive thyroid developed during pregnancy.

Gestational hypothyroidism (underactive thyroid gland). An underactive thyroid gland developed during pregnancy.

Goitre. An enlarged thyroid gland.

Goitrogens. Substances that can block thyroid hormone formation. They can be found in a variety of food including cabbage or other food from the brassica family, where the cabbage falls under.

Graves' disease. An autoimmune thyroid disease that causes hyperthyroidism (overactive thyroid gland).

Graves' ophthalmopathy (GO). Another name for thyroid eye disease.

Hashimoto's disease. Another name for Hashimoto's Thyroiditis.

Hashimoto's thyroiditis. A condition that is the major cause of hypothyroidism. This is also a form of thyroiditis, an autoimmune thyroid disease in which the antibodies attack the thyroid gland, cause it to become infected, then start leaking out its thyroid hormone, and cause the thyroid to shrivel up.

Hashitoxicosis. A condition that is common in the early part of Hashimoto's disease. This condition causes the thyroid hormone to leak out from the gland causing thyrotoxicosis.

High-density lipoprotein (HDL). Good cholesterol. It should be at least 40mg/dl.

Hypercholesterolemia. High cholesterol.

Hypertension. High blood pressure.

Hyperthyroid. An overactive thyroid gland, usually causing thyrotoxicosis.

Hypocalcemia. A condition were the calcium levels are low and can lead to debilitating symptoms.

Hypoparathyroidism. It is when the parathyroid glands do not make sufficient amounts of parathyroid hormone, usually due to damage during thyroid surgery, resulting in hypocalcemia, which can be temporary or permanent.

Hypothalamus. A part of the brain that is just above the pituitary gland, which helps control the pituitary gland and the thyroid gland by releasing the Thyrotropin Releasing Hormone (TRH).

Hypothyroid. Low or nonfunctioning thyroid gland, causing a range of debilitating symptoms associated with low energy and a slowing down of body cells.

I-123. A type of iodine isotope used in thyroid scans.

I-131. A type of iodine isotope used in thyroid scans and treatment.

Iodine. A crucial element the thyroid gland needs to make thyroid hormone.

Iodine deficiency. When not enough iodine from food is available to the thyroid gland; causes hypothyroidism, goitre and, in children or infants, mental retardation, short stature, or cretinism.

Isotope. An element, such as iodine, that is radioactive or unstable.

Isthmus: The middle part of the thyroid gland.

Levethyroxine sodium. Thyroid hormone replacement made by a pharmaceutical company in a pill form. It is also known as L-T4 by physicians and T4 by the public.

Lobectomy. Surgical removal of one lobe of the thyroid gland.

Low-density lipoprotein (LDL). The bad cholesterol. It should be less than 100 mg/dl.

Low-iodine diet. A special diet low in iodine (not sodium) that can maximise the sensitivity and accuracy of radioactive iodine scans or treatments for thyroid cancer.

Lymph nodes: Small nodules containing small white blood cells that stimulate the immune system to fight infection. Cancer cells may grow in lymph nodes, which are removed during the course of thyroid cancer surgery.

Malignant. Cancerous.

Medullary thyroid cancer (MTC). A type of thyroid cancer that can be genetically inherited and treated with surgery if caught early and usually followed up with genetic testing.

Methimazole (Tapazole). An antithyroid medication used to treat hyperthyroidism.

Mild hypothyroidism. Another name for sub-clinical hypothyroidism.

Millicurie. A unit of measurement used for the dosage of radioactive iodine for scans or treatment

MRI. A scan that uses magnetic resonance images.

Neck dissection. A procedure that is performed during thyroidectomy, where the surgeon removes any obvious tumor that has spread to lymph nodes in the neck.

Nodules. Other name for lumps.

Obesity. A body mass index between 30 and 34.9.

Orbital decompression surgery. It is a surgical procedure that removes bone from the eye socket and expands the area alongside the eyeball so that swollen tissue can move into it; Or it can be called a corrective surgery in cases of severe thyroid eye disease.

Osteoporosis. This means bone loss.

Palpitations. A fast and forceful heartbeat.

Panic attack. A cascade of physical symptoms associated with adrenaline and the 'flight or fight' response (feeling nausea and vertigo, cold sweat, chocking sensations, palpitations, and shakiness). Commonly caused by thyrotoxicosis.

Papillary thyroid cancer. A type of thyroid cancer that is usually treatable with surgery and radioactive iodine, with very good outcomes. It accounts for about 80 per cent of all thyroid cancers.

Parathyroid hormone ((PTH). Hormone that causes the kidneys to retain calcium in the blood while releasing phosphorus into the urine. It also increases the activation of vitamin D, which enhances the absorption of calcium and phosphorus from food and beverages.

Pituitary gland. Located in the brain. It acts as a thermostat for the body and makes thyroid-stimulating hormone.

Post-partum thyroiditis. A general label referring to silent thyroiditis occurring after delivery, causing mild hyperthyroidism and short-lived version of Hashimoto's disease.

Propranol. A commonly used beta-blocker.

Proptosis. Protusion, or bulging of the eyeball, associated with thyroid eye disease.

Propylthiouracil (PTU). An antithyroid medication used to treat hyperthyroidism.

Radioactive Iodine (RAI). Iodine that is radioactive; also called an isotope.

RAI. Radioactive iodine.

Riedel's thyroiditis. The rarest form of thyroiditis, in which scar tissue invades the thyroid gland, infiltrates through the gland and binds it to surrounding portions of the neck. It is usually treated with surgery.

Salivary stones. The swelling of one or more salivary glands (located under the ears and under the lower jaw) due to partial blockage of the salivary ducts by dried saliva. These are a complication of radioactive iodine treatment for thyroid cancer.

Silent thyroiditis. A form of thyroiditis so named because it avoids detection until symptoms of thyrotoxicosis (and sometimes hypothyroidism thereafter) become severe. Usually resolves on its own.

Sleep deprivation. Being deprived of the recommended hours of sleep for healthy adults.

Sleep disorder. A physical disorder that interrupts deep, restful sleep. Often not recognised by the sufferer, who may have sleep deprivation.

Stable iodine. Normal, or nonradioactive, iodine.

Subacute viral thyroiditis: Also called de Quervain's thyroiditis. This type of short-lived thyroiditis may be viral in origin. Symptoms are pain and inflammation of the thyroid and thyrotoxicosis for about six weeks.

Subclinical hyperthyroidism. Mild hyperthyroidism with few or no symptoms of thyrotoxicosis.

T3. Short for triiodothyronine.

T4. Short for thyroxine.

Tachycardia. Fast heartbeat (or racing heart). It is associated with hyperthyroidism.

Technetium. A type of isotope used for thyroid scans.

Thyrogen. A pharmaceutically prepared version of thyroid-stimulating hormone made from recombinant DNA technology. It is used in thyroid scans and other tests for thyroid cancer patients.

Thyroglobulin (TG). A protein that is unique to thyroid cells and is the early form of thyroid hormone.

Thyroglobulin test (TG test). A test that measures the amount of thyroglobulin in the blood. It is a useful marker for thyroid cancer cells.

Thyroid antibodies. White blood cells that target the thyroid gland, causing an autoimmune disease.

Thyroid antibody testing. A blood test that checks for the presence of thyroid antibodies.

Thyroidectomy. Surgical removal of the thyroid gland. The procedure can be total or partial.

Thyroid extract. A preparation of dried, cleaned, powdered thyroid glands from cows or pigs. This is also known as natural thyroid hormone.

Thyroid eye disease (TED). An eye disease causing bulging grittiness, redness, double vision, and a range of other eye symptoms, It is also called Graves ophthalmopathy (GO) or Graves' Orbitopathy, and it tends to strike people with Graves' disease.

Thyroid gland. A butterfly-shaped gland typically located in front of the windpipe (trachea) just above the midline bony notch in the top of the breastbone (sternal notch).

Thyroid hormone. A hormone made by the thyroid gland that serves as the speed control for all body cells. Types of thyroid hormone are thyroxine (T4) and triiodothyronine (T3).

Thyroid hormone resistance (Refetoff syndrome). A rare, inherited disease that results in a person being born with a resistance to his or her own thyroid hormone. It is caused by a mutation in the gene that makes the receptors for thyroid hormone.

Thyroiditis. Inflammation of the thyroid gland. Usually causes hypothyroidism.

Thyroid lobe. One side, or lobe, of the thyroid gland. As the gland is butterfly-shaped, a lobe would be one "wing".

Thyroid scan. A test where an image or picture is taken using special cameras and substances that light up for the camera.

Thyroid self-exam. A self-exam of the neck area, which can help find suspicious thyroid lumps or an enlargement of the thyroid gland, which should be evaluated by a doctor.

Thyroid-stimulating hormone (TSH). A special hormone that controls the level of thyroid hormone. High or low TSH levels indicate thyroid function problems.

Thyroid-stimulating immunoglobulin (TSI or TSA). A thyroid antibody that sticks to the thyroid-stimulating hormone receptor instead of to TSH. Overstimulating the thyroid causes Graves' disease or, when sticking to parts of the eye muscle, causes thyroid eye disease.

Thyroid storm. When symptoms of severe thyrotoxicosis can manifest into a storm of severe cardiovascular symptoms that warrant emergency attention and admission to an intensive care unit.

Thyrotoxic. Describes someone who suffers from thyrotoxicosis

Thyrotoxic Goitre. Goitres associated with prolonged thyrotoxicosis caused by Graves' disease or autonomous toxic nodules.

Thyrotoxicosis. Too much thyroid hormone caused by hyperthyroidism. Overdose of thyroid hormone replacement, autonomous toxic nodules, and other types of thyroid conditions lead to a range of debilitating symptoms associated with over-stressed, exhausted body cells causing a speeding up of bodily processes.

Thyrotropin-releasing hormone (TRH). A hormone made by the hypothalamus when thyroid hormone levels are low.

Thyroxine (T4). The inactive form of thyroid hormone. It is called T4 because it contains four iodine atoms for each hormone molecule.

Total T3 test. The appropriate blood test to measure the amount of active thyroid hormone, or T3, levels.

Toxic multinodular Goitre. When the thyroid gland forms multiple nodules that produces too much thyroid hormone.

Triiodothyronine (T3). Made by the body's cells out of T4. This is the active thyroid hormone that activates genes and "does the job" of the thyroid hormone.

TSH. Thyroid-stimulating hormone.

TSH test. A sensitive blood test that assesses whether thyroid-stimulating hormone levels are high or low by looking at the body's own natural "thermostat" for thyroid hormone.

Ultrasound. A device that uses high-frequency sound waves to produce an "echo picture" of a structure in the body.

Undifferentiated thyroid cancer cells. Cancer cells that do not retain the functional features of normal thyroid follicular cells.

Unipolar depression. The most common type of depression, characterised by one low, flat mood. It is frequently a complication of hypothyroidism.

WBS. Whole body scan.

Whole body scan (WBS). It is a scan that involve pictures of the whole body which are used to track the thyroid cancer recurrence

www.ingramcontent.com/pod-product-compliance
Lightning Source LLC
Chambersburg PA
CBHW020356290526
45785CB00005B/2306